AROMATHERAPY

the essential blending guide

Bev Wishes

Rosemary Caddy

Creating a collection of pure medicinal blends for common ailments

Rosemary Caddy

BSc ARCS MISPA

Amberwood Publishing Ltd
Rochester - England
Phone: (01634) 290115   Fax: (01634) 290761
E-mail: books@amberwoodpublishing.com
Website: www.amberwoodpublishing.com

© Amberwood Publishing Ltd 2000

First Edition June 2000
Second Edition August 2002
Third Edition January 2007

ISBN 1-899308-24-5

 Design and Typeset by C.C.Profiles

Cover design by Howland Northover & Rosemary Caddy

Printed in Great Britain

Contents

About the Author

Rosemary Caddy, BSc Hons, ARCS, MISPA

Rosemary Caddy graduated from London University with a BSc Honours Degree in Science. As a Reader and Principal Lecturer in Educational Research at Nottingham University she is the author of a range of educational materials for students of many disciplines. All the materials emphasise visual presentation to enable students to see, analyse and understand the world around them. The format of this work ranges from books to interactive video tapes and compact discs.

Rosemary is now a qualified clinical aromatherapist running her own clinic and carrying out a programme of research on the chemistry of essential oils. She runs lecture courses for aromatherapy students to help them understand and visualise their essential oils. The Caddy Classic Profiles, developed as a result of her research enable students to enjoy the chemistry of their oils.

Currently Rosemary is researching the chemistry of synergistic mixes of essential oils.

Note to Reader

Whilst the author has made every effort to ensure that the contents of this book are accurate in every particular, it is not intended to be regarded as a substitute for professional medical advice under treatment. The reader is urged to give careful consideration to any difficulties which he or she is experiencing with their own health and to consult their General Practitioner if uncertain as to its cause or nature. Neither the author nor the publisher can accept any legal responsibility for any health problem which results from the use of the self-help methods described.

Acknowledgements

My interest in essential oils derives from personal experience of their powerful therapeutic properties, both in treating physical ailments and also in calming emotional problems.

Exploring the chemistry of essential oils gives some insights as to why the oils are so powerful.

My background in lecturing and research has been focused on using strong visual stimuli to communicate complex structures. Colour and pictures are excellent learning aids. Caddy Classic Profiles have been created to help communicate the nature of essential oils.

They first appeared in the book 'Essential Oils in Colour'. I would like to thank the many students and colleagues who have kindly written in appreciation of the book. With their encouragement this book 'The Essential Blending Guide', the CD 'The Caddy Blending Calculator' and the Caddy Training Packs have been developed. Thanks are also expressed to Katja Svoboda and her team at The Scottish Agricultural College for assistance in research into essential oils and their synergistic mixes.

It has again been a privilege to work with June Crisp and the Amberwood publishing team.

I would also like to thank all my friends, family, colleagues and students who listen to all my enthusiasms so patiently. In particular special thanks to Peter, my husband, for his unflagging support, valuable suggestions and for once again his painstaking editing of manuscript and indices.

My appreciation also goes to the services of Nottingham and Exeter University Libraries , The British Library, The Royal Horticultural Society, Oxford Botanical Gardens and to my own local Dartmouth Library.

Welcome

Essential Oils in the home can herald a new way of life. These wonderful natural plant products can play a vital role in both our physical and mental well being. Many books have been written detailing the therapeutic properties of essential oils. This book offers very practical advice on how to use the oils in the home and how to create your own

Home Collection

One well tested *BLEND* recipe is given for each Common Ailment. Rather like a basic cookery book you can regard the recipes for each Common Ailment as a basic recipe that you can rely on. As you become more familiar with your essential oils you can explore *BLENDS* of your own. (see Appendix - Caddy Blending Calculator) As you make up each *BLEND* your Home Collection will become well stocked. You will be gradually introduced to all the essential oils by experiencing them in action.

——Common Ailments List——

Common Ailments List

	page
Gastric Flatulence	74
Gout	76
Haemorrhoids	78
Headaches	80
Herpes Simplex	82
Impetigo	84
Indigestion	86
Leg Ulcers	88
Measles	90
Menopause	92
Mumps	94
Osteoarthritis	96
Periods - heavy	98
Periods - lack of	100
Periods - painful	102
Periods - pmt	104
Post-natal Infections	106
Rheumatoid Arthritis	108
Ringworm	110
Sex Drive Problems	112
Sprains	114
Stretch Marks	116
Thrush	118
Varicose Veins	120
Weight Loss	122

How to Use this Book

title of Common Ailment pages 24 to 123

key to the chemical families gives the percentage of each chemical family in the blend page 22

pie chart showing the percentage of each chemical family in the blend this is called the Caddy Classic Profile of the blend (CCP of blend) page 22

blend recipe gives the ratio in which the oils are mixed as shown by the drops. For this blend the ratio is 2:1:1 page 18

the small pie charts are the Caddy Classic Profiles (CCP) of the individual oils page 22

therapeutic properties of each individual oil used in the blend

key to the chemical constituents in the blend page 22

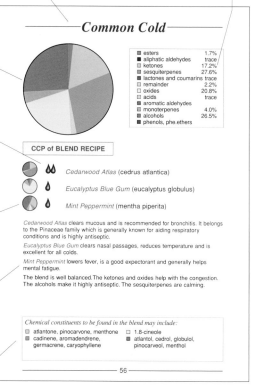

Common Cold

■ esters	1.7%
■ aliphatic aldehydes	trace
☐ ketones	17.2%
■ sesquiterpenes	27.6%
■ lactones and coumarins	trace
☐ remainder	2.2%
☐ oxides	20.8%
☐ acids	trace
■ aromatic aldehydes	
■ monoterpenes	4.0%
■ alcohols	26.5%
■ phenols, phe.ethers	

CCP of BLEND RECIPE

♨♨ *Cedarwood Atlas* (cedrus atlantica)

♨ *Eucalyptus Blue Gum* (eucalyptus globulus)

♨ *Mint Peppermint* (mentha piperita)

Cedarwood Atlas clears mucous and is recommended for bronchitis. It belongs to the Pinaceae family which is generally known for aiding respiratory conditions and is highly antiseptic.

Eucalyptus Blue Gum clears nasal passages, reduces temperature and is excellent for all colds.

Mint Peppermint lowers fever, is a good expectorant and generally helps mental fatigue.

The blend is well balanced. The ketones and oxides help with the congestion. The alcohols make it highly antiseptic. The sesquiterpenes are calming.

Chemical constituents to be found in the blend may include:

☐ atlantone, pinocarvone, menthone   ☐ 1.8-cineole
■ cadinene, aromadendrene,   ■ atlantol, cedrol, globulol,
   germacrene, caryophyllene   pinocarveol, menthol

— 56 —

Detailed information of all the essential oils used to make the blends in this book can be found in the book called
'Essential Oils in Colour' ISBN 1-899308-14-8 (see Appendix).
The full therapeutic properties of 90 oils, as reported from professional aromatherapists, are given together with full size Caddy Classic Profiles showing the chemical make-up of the oils.

blend for your
HOME COLLECTION
pages 20 to 21

BLEND

20 drops *Cedarwood Atlas*
10 drops *Eucalyptus Blue Gum*
10 drops *Mint Peppermint*
40 drops BLEND

Make up your BLEND using the quantities above - store in a small dark glass bottle fitted with a dropper (see page 20).

GARGLE

A *Teatree* oil gargle is helpful at the onset of all colds especially if a sore throat is a symptom.
Add 1 drop of *Teatree* (melaleuca alternifolia) oil to a glass of warm boiled water.
Gargle at frequent intervals.

MASSAGE

Add 12 drops of the BLEND to 30ml of Sweet Almond Oil to make up a supply of Common Cold Treatment Oil (see page 20).
Alternatively add 12 drops of the BLEND to 30ml of body cream or lotion
Massage chest, neck and upper back areas morning and night.
Concentrate thumb massage around the vertebrae as this stimulates the action of the oils.
A facial massage with this Treatment Oil helps sinusitis sufferers.
Rub a small amount of Treatment Oil under the nostrils when going to bed.

ROOM SPRAY

Add 12 drops of the BLEND to 1 litre of water. Spray freely in any room.

TISSUES

Place 2 to 4 drops of the BLEND onto a paper tissue.
Wrap the tissue in foil and pop it in your pocket so that you can inhale the vapours from the tissue at regular intervals during the day.
To ease congestion at night place such a tissue on the soles of your feet. The vapour from the oils passes around the body as you sleep.

VAPOURISER

Place 4 to 6 drops of the BLEND in the vapouriser.
It helps to keep the vapouriser going in any room where you are spending any length of time.
This also guards against others contracting your condition.

BATHS

Place 8 drops of the BLEND into a warm bath.
Relax and inhale the vapours.
This is particularly helpful before going to bed.

DIET

Two or three garlic tablets each day are recommended.
Cut down on all dairy food as this encourages the production of mucous in the system.
Take regular doses of vitamin C tablets or drinks.
Follow a light healthy diet of fruit and vegetables.

the various methods for home use, relevant for the Ailment, are listed - detailed notes on all the methods of using essential oils and blends are given on pages 13 to 17

Using the Common Cold as an example you can see how all the information for each Common Ailment is presented (see pages 24 to123).

For more details on each part of the information refer to the pages referenced against each section.

Before starting to use the blends and treatments take time to read through the pages preceding the Common Ailments as you will find useful detailed information and definitions.

Getting Started

One of the easiest ways to meet the different essential oils is to use a vaporiser like the ones shown above. All you need to do is to place water in the top of the vapouriser and add a few drops of essential oil to it. Light the candle and you soon smell the aroma of your oil.

How Essential Oils Work

The electrochemical nature of essential oil molecules is such that they tend to release charged particles when placed in water. Once the molecules enter our blood stream this electrochemical property comes into play. Travelling to all parts of the body it is believed that the essential oil molecules help the body to correct and maintain a healthy electrochemical balance. This is one of the ways that essential oils strengthen the body's natural healing powers.

Building up your Essential Oils

It takes a while to build up a complete stock of essential oils. Start off with just purchasing the ones that you need for a specific ailment. Make sure that you store them in a dry dark cupboard and then they will have a shelf life of 2 to 3 years.

A possible strategy to help with the cost is to find 2 or 3 friends who are willing to buy the essential oils together. This can be the common stock from which you each make up your own Common Ailment *BLENDS*

The *BLENDS* only require a few drops of each essential oil so sharing the essential oils makes good sense.

Read the treatment information carefully and always use the quantities given.

Using Essential Oils

*E*ssential oils are one of nature's kindest gifts. Their wonderful range of aromas can help every mood and feeling. Their therapeutic powers are remarkable and they provide us with the means to build a home collection that is a present from the plants around us.

Essential oils contain many chemical constituents that are manufactured by the plants during their growth cycles. Plants store their essential oils in different places. The geranium has its oil stored in its leaves. You only need to crush a geranium leaf to smell the aroma. Pine trees store their essential oil in their needles. If you walk through a wood of pine trees you will smell the essential oil molecules as they evaporate from the needles. A stroll through such a place is a natural tonic for our lungs. All essential oils are volatile and will evaporate sharing their molecules and aromas. Just a few drops of rose will scent a whole room.

Breathing in the scent from an essential oil means that thousands of the oil's molecules will find their way into your blood stream and be carried to all parts of your body. These special molecules help the body's healing processes in a gentle but effective fashion.

There are many ways in which we can ensure that the essential oil molecules reach our blood stream. The most commonly used ways are listed here and can all be quite easily organised in the home.

VAPOURISERS

You can purchase these from chemists and health shops, they are widely available. The major part of a vapouriser is the bowl at the top. This you fill with water. Under the bowl is some means of heating the water - usually a night light candle but vapourisers with electric heaters are also available. You place a few drops of essential oil in the water. As the water is heated the essential oil is heated and its molecules evaporate into the room filling it with a wonderful aroma. It is wise to choose a vapouriser with a sensible size of bowl so that you get a maximum time of evaporation before it runs 'dry'.

This method of using essential oils is one of the simplest and also extremely effective:

an essential oil such as *Bergamot* relieves anxiety;

an essential oil such as *Tea Tree* inhibits infection by airborne bacteria;

an essential oil such as *Eucalyptus* helps to clear congestion;

an essential oil such as *Lavender* helps combat insomnia and so on.

As you meet the essential oils and their *BLENDS* you can try many different combinations in your vapouriser. They are great fun for festive occasions. For example the scent of *Cinnamon* wafting through the house at Christmas time is warm and welcoming.

TISSUES

This is another simple method - you just take a paper tissue and put 2 to 3 drops of essential oil onto it. You then inhale deeply 2 or 3 times and your nose and nasal passages fill with essential oil molecules. *Eucalyptus* oils are particularly effective in clearing nasal congestion.

A tip for cold sufferers is to prepare a tissue for use in this way then wrap it in foil and pop it in a pocket for use during the day. The tissue technique is also useful if you are anxious and tense. *Bergamot* oil can be extremely helpful in controlling panic attacks.

CAR VAPOURISERS

These are small unglazed porcelain containers. You simply drop 8 to 10 drops of essential oil into the container. The molecules evaporate through the porcelain and the aroma wafts through the car.
An essential oil such as *Rosemary* alleviates fatigue and *Peppermint* helps with car sickness.

BATHS

To use essential oils in your bath is a simple process. Run your bath as normal then simply sprinkle 6 to 8 drops of essential oil into the bath. Swish the water around to disperse the oil.
Lie in the bath for a minimum of 15 minutes. The warmth of the water helps the skin to absorb the molecules of essential oil. So with this method the oils are being inhaled through the nasal passages and being absorbed through the skin.
It is safe to use this method everyday. As you explore essential oils you will find combinations which will help your moods and ailments. Some people prefer to add the essential oils to a special carrier base first. The special carrier base helps to disperse the essential oil in the water. You can purchase the special carrier base from an essential oil supplier. However if you choose to add the individual drops of essential oil directly you can vary your bath to suit your mood.

COMPRESSES

Cut a piece of clean cotton sheeting to the required size. Prepare a bowl of water by adding a few drops of essential oil.
Use hot water for muscular aches and cold water for sprains, bruises or headaches. Soak the cotton sheeting in the water and oil, wring out, and apply gently to the required area. Cover with cling film and leave in place for a while. A compress is a well tested technique for helping swelling, bruising, sprains and aches. It is also a gentle way to get fragile skin to absorb the essential oils.

MOUTH WASHES AND GARGLES

Use 1 drop of *Tea Tree* oil to a glassful of water. Rinse the mouth or gargle with the mix spitting it out afterwards. This treatment can relieve inflamed surfaces in the mouth and help with mouth ulcers. Essential oils have good antiseptic properties so this treatment will help fight infection.

ROOM SPRAY

Fill an indoor plant spray with boiled water add a few drops of essential oil and you have a room spray. Spray throughout the house and the molecules of essential oil will be a natural sweet smelling antiseptic. An ideal way to keep infection at bay.

WATER SPRAY

It can be helpful to spray a very delicate area such as a leg ulcer with a fine spray of water containing essential oil molecules. This creates an antiseptic barrier around the wound as well as helping to heal the wound. To use this method you require a small water spray bottle that you can purchase from a chemist. Prepare a small cup of warm boiled water and add 2 drops of the chosen essential oils to it. Spray the required area according to directions. Always make up the water mixture freshly each day.

CREAM APPLICATION

You can make up a jar of cream not only to help with specific skin problems but also to help with other ailments. For each ailment cream you choose a suitable *BLEND* of essential oils. Typically you add 12 drops of your *BLEND* to 30ml of unmedicated body cream. This cream can be gently massaged into the required area. *Tea Tree* cream is a useful one to make up to treat Athlete's Foot.

SHAMPOO

You can purchase bottles of shampoo base from essential oil suppliers. Add a few drops of your favourite essential oils and you have a personal shampoo.

MASSAGE

To make up a massage oil you add in the order of 12 drops of essential oil to 30ml of Carrier Oil. Exact quantities are given for treatments in the book. Be sure to follow all the directions carefully. A professional aromatherapist has the expertise to massage the body such that the muscles relax and the blood and lymph flow freely around the body. This enhances the body's immune system and stimulates the body's natural healing powers. The power of relaxation plays a large part in the body's well being.
You can, yourself, bring considerable relief to some conditions by gentle massage on affected areas. The hands and feet in particular respond well to gentle rubbing with a massage oil.

Cedarwood Atlas — 2 drops

Eucalyptus Blue Gum — 1 drop

Mint Peppermint — 1 drop

Common Cold BLEND — 4 drops

Common Cold BLEND

Whenever the word *BLEND* is used in this book it means a *BLEND* of essential oils that has not been diluted with a carrier oil.

A carrier oil that has some drops of *BLEND* added to it is always called a Treatment Oil.

This book provides you with the recipes for 50 *BLENDS* of essential oils that have proved very powerful in treating common ailments. As your collection of essential oils and *BLENDS* grows you will become familiar with the nature of the individual essential oils.

For every common ailment *BLEND* relevant therapeutic notes for the essential oils in its recipe are given.

For every common ailment *BLEND* its chemical constituents are given and the Caddy Classic Profile (see page 22) shows the chemical families in the *BLEND*.

For every common ailment full treatment notes are given which are easy to use in the home.

Carriers

Carrier oils are non volatile oils that are used for making up Treatment Oils that can be massaged or applied to the skin. You may like to buy a range of carrier oils to use when you make up your Treatment Oils as they also offer benefits to the body. Here are some brief notes to help you.

Grapeseed Oil

This in its natural state can be dark in colour with a strong odour. To make it usable it is often highly refined which renders it less beneficial. However it is widely used and reasonably priced.

Sweet Almond Oil

This is a mild neutral oil used widely for massage.

Sunflower Oil

Virgin, cold pressed, sunflower oil is an economic, neutral oil. It has an affinity to human sebum and is a good baby oil.

Walnut Oil

Virgin walnut oil is highly recommended as an all round massage oil. It is high in unsaturated fatty acids, particularly GLA.

Jojoba Oil

This is semi wax-like when cold. Contains vitamin E and has excellent skin softening qualities.

Calendula Oil

This is a macerated oil. It is excellent for skin care and will be added to a main carrier oil rather than used on its own. For example in making up a Treatment Oil you might use 25ml of sweet almond oil with 5 ml of calendula oil as your carrier oils.

St. John's Wort (Hypericum) Oil

Again a macerated oil which has been used since ancient times in many remedies. It is blood red in colour and helps with anxiety states and relaxes muscles. When making up a Treatment Oil you could use 29ml of walnut oil with 1ml of St John's Wort oil as your carrier oils.

Other bases used as carriers for the *BLENDS* include

White Carrier Lotion

This is a non oily carrier that will not stain clothing - an alternative to the carrier oils but less rich in therapeutic benefits.

Cream Bases

Various base creams can be purchased from essential oil suppliers and chemists. Check details with the suppliers.

Shampoo and Bath Base Carriers

These can also be purchased from essential oil suppliers. With these you can make up your own bath and shampoo mixtures.

*E*ssential oils come in coloured glass bottles that are fitted with dropper attachments. When you order essential oils - order some empty bottles to store your *BLENDS* in. The 7ml bottles will be plenty large enough. For Example:-

To make up the Common Cold *BLEND* you need
20 drops of *Cedarwood Atlas* (cedrus atlantica)
10 drops of *Eucalyptus Blue Gum* (eucalyptus globulus)
10 drops of *Mint Peppermint* (mentha piperita)
Ease the dropper attachment out of your 7ml bottle. Add the correct number of drops of each oil to the bottle. Replace the dropper and screw the lid on firmly.

Prepare a label something like the one shown below.

Home Collection 56	blend ratio
Common Cold	2 of cedrus atlantica
	1 of eucalyptus globulus
BLEND	1 of mentha piperita

You have made up 40 drops of Common Cold *BLEND* which is about 2ml of *BLEND*. You can add this to the stock in your

Home Collection

You can always make up smaller or larger quantities - just keep the ratio of the essential oils the same as the recipe. In the Common Cold *BLEND* the ratio is 2 drops of *Cedarwood* to 1 drop of *Eucalytptus* to 1 drop of *Peppermint*.

Essential oils will keep well if you store them in a dry dark cupboard. Your *BLENDS* will have a shelf life of 2 to 3 years.

Once you have prepared your Ailment *BLEND* you can add drops of it to a bath, to a vapouriser, to water sprays and so on, as directed for each ailment.

Treatment Oil and Treatment Cream

If an Ailment requires a massage treatment or a skin application treatment you need to make up a Treatment Oil or a Treatment Cream as directed.

To make up a Treatment Oil you need a 30ml glass bottle as shown above. The 30ml bottle should not have a dropper attachment. If it has remove it and do not replace it.
To make up a Treatment Oil fill a 30ml bottle with a carrier oil (see page 19) and add the specified number of Ailment *BLEND* drops.
A prepared Treatment Oil will store for 2 to 3 weeks. Normally you will have used it all before then.

To make up a Treatment Cream fill a 30ml pot with a base cream (see page 19) and add the specified number of Ailment *BLEND* drops. Mix thoroughly with a spatula.
A prepared Treatment Cream will store for 5 to 6 months.

Label your treatment bottles and pots clearly.
You can purchase your bottles, pots, carrier oils and cream from your essential oil supplier. Other carrier lotions and ointments that are needed for the Ailments can be purchased from the chemist.

*E*ach essential oil has its own aroma and its own unique chemical make-up. There are many books that detail the reported therapeutic properties of each oil and these reports are a good guide when deciding which oils will help a specific condition.

The book 'Essential Oils in Colour' (see back pages) lists the reported therapeutic properties of all the oils that are used in this book. It also illustrates the chemical make-up of each oil by a brightly coloured piechart called a Caddy Classic Profile (CCP). This chart shows the amount of each of the major chemical families that are typically present in each essential oil. They provide a clear fingerprint for each oil that conveys the chemical nature of the oil. In this book we show the CCP for each *BLEND* of essential oils.

Major Chemical Families

Here we give a brief description of the chemical families that are shown in a CCP. The table below shows the colour coding used in a CCP and lists a few of the possible therapeutic properties that the chemical families may contribute to an essential oil.

esters	calming good for skin problems
aliphatic aldehydes	refreshing, antiseptic, antifungal
ketones	cooling, decongestant, analgesic
sesquiterpenes	balancing, soothing, digestion, warming
lactones.& coumarins	balancing, decongestant, photosensitive
remainder	the unreported part of the oil i.e, the remainder
oxides	expectorant, respiratory decongestant, diuretic
acids	deodourant, present in very small quantities
aromatic aldehydes	warming, antiseptic, antifungal
monoterpenes	skin tonic, digestion, liver
alcohols	antiviral, bactericidal, tonic but gentle
phenols, phe.ethers	stimulating, antiviral, aggressive

If you see a large amount of the ester blue colour you know that the oil is rich in esters. This alerts you to the fact that this oil may well help skin conditions so you check its reported properties to see if that is indeed so.

If you see a large amount of the light blue ketone colour, showing that the oil is rich in ketones, you are alerted to the fact that caution may be required in the use of this oil as ketones can accumulate in the body. Again check the properties of the oil to see if this is so.

An alert is also given when you see a large area of the dark red showing that the oil is rich in phenols. This chemical family can be highly aggressive so once more check the properties of the oil as reported in the literature.

Alcohols and esters are nearly always safe and gentle in use. Thus knowing the chemical make-up of an oils alerts you to possibilities for its therapeutic properties. However you must always refer to the reported properties of the oil to check out these possibilities. This is because each essential oil is unique in its chemical make-up. The particular set of molecules present forms the whole oil and it is the property of the whole oil that is important.

The Caddy Classic Profile (CCP)

The CCP gives the typical chemical nature of an oil at a glance and allows you to quickly compare it with other essential oils.

Imagine that a chemist reports that he has found an essential oil that is really remarkable in that it typically contains all the chemical families and each one is 8% of the oil. Its CCP would be:

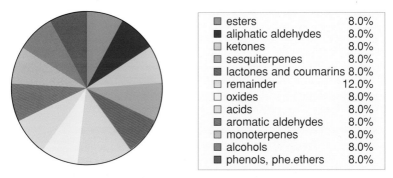

☐ esters	8.0%
■ aliphatic aldehydes	8.0%
☐ ketones	8.0%
☐ sesquiterpenes	8.0%
■ lactones and coumarins	8.0%
☐ remainder	12.0%
☐ oxides	8.0%
☐ acids	8.0%
■ aromatic aldehydes	8.0%
▨ monoterpenes	8.0%
▨ alcohols	8.0%
■ phenols, phe.ethers	8.0%

When an oil is analysed it is expensive to identify every single chemical constituent - usually an oil distributor requests identification of the most important chemicals. The chemist in this example has identified 88% of the oil so there is still 12% of the oil's chemical constituents unidentified. This 12% remainder is shown in light green. The colours used in the CCP's give you an immediate view of the electrochemical nature of each *BLEND*. The 'blue' families share a molecular structure such that they generate negatively charged particles and the 'yellow to red' families share a molecular structure such that they generate positive particles. This tends to show up in the fact that except for a few exceptions *BLENDS* with large areas of 'blues' tend to be more relaxing, those with large areas of 'yellows to reds' tend to be more stimulating and the 'greens' are more associated with balancing properties.

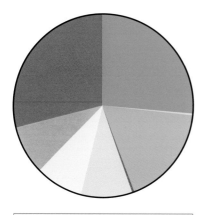

☐ esters	26.2%
■ aliphatic aldehydes	trace
☐ ketones	0.1%
☐ sesquiterpenes	18.5%
■ lactones and coumarins	0.2%
☐ remainder	9.0%
☐ oxides	8.6%
☐ acids	trace
■ aromatic aldehydes	trace
☐ monoterpenes	8.0%
☐ alcohols	29.4%
■ phenols, phe.ethers	trace

CCP of BLEND RECIPE

  Orange Petitgrain (citrus aurantium amara)

  Chamomile Maroc (ormenis multicaulis)

  Niaouli (melaleuca viridiflora)

  Cedar Virginian Red (juniperus virginiana)

Orange Petitgrain is a strongly bactericidal and is also a calming and cheering oil. It recommended to treat infected acne. The aroma is woody and floral.

Chamomile Maroc is an effective antiseptic, decongestant and bactericidal. It is recommended for eczema, dry cracked skin, infected pus and acne.

Niaouli is highly antiseptic and tones and heals skin conditions including acne, boils, spots and ulcers.

Cedar Virginian Red helps to tone oily skin. Treats acne, eczema and dandruff.

Chemical constituents to be found in the blend may include:

- ☐ linalyl acetate, geranyl acetate neryl acetate, bornyl acetate bornyl butyrate
- ☐ β-caryophyllene, bisabolene cedrene, germacrene, thujopsene
- ☐ 1.8-cineole
- ☐ α-pinene, β-pinene, myrcene limonene
- ■ linalool, geraniol, α-terpineol santolina alcohol, yomogi alcohol, artemisia alcohol, viridiflorol, cedrol, globulol, widdrol, γ-eudesmol.

BLEND

18drops *Orange Petitgrain*
 6 drops *Chamomile Maroc*
 6 drops *Niaouli*
12 drops *Cedar Virginia Red*
42 drops *BLEND*

Make up your *BLEND* using the quantities above - store in a small dark glass bottle fitted with a dropper (see page 20).

AILMENT

Acne is caused by abnormal activity of the sebaceous glands which results in over production of sebum. This blocks the hair pores with a greasy plug. These sometimes show up as blackheads. Sebaceous glands appear to be affected by hormonal changes and stress, which can also trigger hormonal changes in the body. This is why acne is extremely common during puberty.

It is vital not to squeeze or damage the skin around affected areas as this can cause bacterial infection to become worse. This is when scarring occurs.

The *BLEND* treatments will help combat the bacterial infection and encourage the skin to heal.

The diet suggestions are aimed at encouraging the body to achieve a hormonal balance to stop the sebaceous glands over producing sebum.

It will take several months for the condition to improve so patience and perseverance is needed.

Do not use sunbeds and although sunlight will help do not over expose the skin as this can make the condition worse.

SKIN APPLICATIONS

Make up a bottle of Acne Treatment Oil by adding 12 drops of *BLEND* to 30ml of Jojoba Oil and 5ml of Calendula Oil (see Carriers).

Also make up a bottle of Acne Treatment Lotion by adding 12 drops of *BLEND* to 30ml of lotion.

Every night, sparingly apply the Acne Treatment Oil to the affected areas.

Each morning sparingly apply the Acne Treatment Lotion to the affected areas.

For treatment during the day prepare cotton wool pads in the following way. Add 5 drops of *BLEND* to half a cup of spring water. Soak cotton wool pads in the water then squeeze them out and put into a small plastic bag. Gently wipe the affected skin with these pads every two hours.

Following these instructions will keep the skin protected from infection for the full 24 hours.

BATHS

Add 8 drops of *BLEND* to your baths.

DIET

Eat plenty of vegetables but only a modest amount of fruit. Avoid fatty foods, dairy foods and red meat as much as possible. Drink 7 glasses of water a day.

Daily Supplements
Vitamin A dose as stated on container
Vitamin C 1000 mgs
Zinc 30-40 mgs
Vitamin E 600 mgs

esters	39.0%
aliphatic aldehydes	0.6%
ketones	trace
sesquiterpenes	0.4%
lactones and coumarins	2.6%
remainder	4.9%
oxides	0.1%
acids	trace
aromatic aldehydes	
monoterpenes	23.2%
alcohols	29.0%
phenols, phe.ethers	0.2%

CCP of BLEND RECIPE

 𝄞𝄞𝄞 *Bergamot* (citrus bergamia)

 𝄞𝄞 *Orange Petitgrain* (citrus aurantium amara)

 𝄞 *Rose Otto* (rosa damascena)

Bergamot is antispasmodic and calming. It is excellent for agitation and panic attacks. It is often the first choice in cases of depression. The aroma is light and citrus.

Orange Petitgrain is antispasmodic, calming and cheering. It is recommended in cases of nervous exhaustion. It also stimulates the immune system. The aroma is woody and floral.

Rose Otto calms anxiety. It has a sweet heavenly flowery aroma that lingers in the room. It relieves tension and feelings of inadequancy.

This blend of essential oils is particularly useful in relieving anxiety and tension. The strong aroma from *Rose Otto* is due to the damascenone.

Chemical constituents to be found in the blend may include:

- linalyl acetate, geranyl acetate neryl acetate
- citral
- damascenone
- rose oxide

- α-pinene, β-pinene, γ-terpinene α–terpinene, myrcene, limonene stearoptene
- linalool, geraniol, α-terpineol, nerol, citronellol, phenylethyl alcohol

BLEND

21 drops	*Bergamot*
14 drops	*Orange Petitgrain*
7 drops	*Rose Otto*
42 drops	*BLEND*

Make up your *BLEND* using the quantities above - store in a small dark glass bottle fitted with a dropper (see page 20).

AILMENT

Continued anxiety upsets the balance between the various body functions. Conditions such as stomach ulcers and heart disease can be the result of unrelieved anxiety. A common physical symptom of anxiety is excess muscle tension. Massage treatment with the *BLEND* eases muscle tension and helps to calm anxious feelings.

It is important to identify and tackle the cause of the anxiety. A table showing the most common causes of stress and anxiety is given in the Appendix.

MASSAGE

Make up a bottle of Anxiety Treatment Oil by adding 12 drops of *BLEND* to 30ml of Sweet Almond Oil. (see page 20)

Take time to rest quietly and gently massage the treatment oil around your shoulders and neck. Even better lie face down on a couch and ask a friend or partner to gently massage your back. Another very good way to get relaxed is to simply have your feet gently rubbed or massaged with the Treatment Oil.

For real help in a case of chronic anxiety seek the professional help of an aromatherapist or reflexologist.

BATHS

Add 8 drops of *BLEND* to your baths.

VAPOURISERS

Add 5 drops of *BLEND* or 5 drops of Bergamot to a vapouriser. This is particularly helpful at night or on any occasion when anxiety threatens to cause a panic attack.

TISSUE

Sprinkle 5 drops of *BLEND* onto a tissue. Wrap this up and keep in a pocket. Use it to inhale deeply whenever necessary.

LIFE STYLE

Lack of fresh air, exercise and poor working conditions can lead to mental fatigue. Try to find time for outdoor activities. A daily walk can be really helpful. Relaxation, meditation and yoga are recommended. Also try to find a 'laugh' a day.

DIET

Follow a balanced diet with plenty of fruit and vegetables. Avoid tea and coffee and any drinks with tannin in them.

Daily Supplements
Vitamin B Complex as directed on the container
Vitamin C 250 - 500mgs

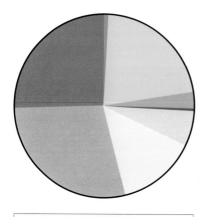

☐ esters	0.7%
■ aliphatic aldehydes	
☐ ketones	21.7%
☐ sesquiterpenes	3.0%
■ lactones and coumarins	0.1%
☐ remainder	6.6%
☐ oxides	13.6%
☐ acids	trace
■ aromatic aldehydes	
☐ monoterpenes	28.6%
☐ alcohols	25.7%
■ phenols, phe.ethers	

CCP of BLEND RECIPE

  Lavender Spike (lavandula lactifolia)

  Tea Tree (melaleuca alternifolia)

  Tagetes (tagetes glandulifera)

Lavender Spike is antifungal and in general helpful with skin problems such as athlete's foot and ringworm.

Tea Tree is strongly antiseptic which helps to protect any skin wounds from infection. Recommended for boils, bites, cold sores, sweaty feet, athlete's foot and mouth ulcers.

Tagetes as well as helping athlete's foot to clear it is also useful for bunions, callouses and tired feet in general.

The ketones and alcohols will offer antifungal properties to this blend. The blend of the three oils attacks the condition and keeps the area free of infection.

Chemical constituents to be found in the blend may include:

☐ linalyl acetate
☐ tagetone, tagetenones, camphor
☐ 1.8-cineole

☐ α-pinene, γ-terpinene
limonene, α-terpinene, ocimene
terpinolene, *p*-cymene
■ terpinen-4-ol, α-terpineol, linalool

BLEND

15 drops *Lavender Spike*
15 drops *Tea Tree*
15 drops *Tagetes*
45 drops *BLEND*

Make up your *BLEND* using the quantities above - store in a small dark glass bottle fitted with a dropper (see page 20).

AILMENT

Athlete's foot is the common name for a type of ringworm that infects the feet. The skin between the toes especially between the outer toes becomes infected with a microscopic fungus. It gets its name from the fact that it is often picked up in changing rooms of schools and sports clubs. The infected skin becomes thickened and moist. Eventually the skin becomes itchy and dries leading to cracking and peeling.

LIFE STYLE

Always dry your feet thoroughly especially between the toes. Change socks and tights frequently. In fact if possible only wear cotton or wool garments.

POWDER

Add 3 drops of the *BLEND* to a cup of talc. Mix it well. An electric blender with a fitted lid is ideal for this job. Powder the feet every day and place a little powder in all your footware.

FOOT BATHS

Add 6 drops of *BLEND* to a bowl of warm water and soak feet every day. Dry well afterwards, particularly between the toes.

APPLICATION

Make up a bottle of Athlete's Foot Treatment Oil by adding 4 drops of *BLEND* to 30ml of Grapeseed Oil. Massage the feet with the Treatment Oil every night before going to bed. Make up a pot of Athlete's Foot Treatment Cream by adding 4 drops of *BLEND* to 30ml of body and hand cream. Keep this Treatment Cream in the cupboard and use as a preventative measure. Apply to feet after visiting any place where you are likely to pick up the infection. In particular after visiting swimming pools and changing rooms.

Baby Colic

☐ esters	38.5%
■ aliphatic aldehydes	1.5%
☐ ketones	1.5%
☐ sesquiterpenes	3.0%
■ lactones and coumarins	trace
☐ remainder	3.0%
☐ oxides	2.5%
☐ acids	trace
■ aromatic aldehydes	
▨ monoterpenes	22.5%
☐ alcohols	27.5%
■ phenols, phe.ethers	trace

CCP of BLEND RECIPE

  Chamomile Roman (chamaemelum nobile)

  Marjoram Sweet (origanum majorana)

Chamomile Roman is a member of the compositae botanical family which is known to be generally soothing to the skin and calming to the digestive system. This oil is antispasmodic and calming. It is recommended for intestinal colic, flatulence and is helpful for jaundice and liver conditions. The aroma is fruity and apple like. This oil is an excellent oil for use with babies.

Marjoram Sweet has a spicy warm camphor like aroma. It is helpful in treating diarrhoea, enteritis and flatulence.
It can have powerful effects on hyperactivity being calming to the nervous system.
Known in folklore as 'joy of the mountain' it is associated with bringing peace and tranquillity.

Chemical constituents to be found in the blend may include:

- ▨ linalyl acetate, terpinyl acetate geranyl acetate, angelates, tiglates butyrates
- ■ citral
- ☐ pinocarvone
- ▨ chamazulene, caryophyllene,

- ☐ 1.8-cineole
- ▨ β-pinene, γ-terpinene, α-terpinene limonene, myrcene, ocimene, *p*-cymene, sabinene
- ▨ farnesol, α-terpineol, linalool terpinen-4-ol

BLEND

10 drops	Chamomile Roman
10 drops	Marjoram Sweet
20 drops	BLEND

Make up your BLEND using the quantities above - store in a small dark glass bottle fitted with a dropper (see page 20).

AILMENT

Baby Colic is bouts of stomach pain that commonly affect young babies. It is very worrying to new mothers as the baby is often inconsolable until the griping pain ceases. The pain comes in waves over several hours and can recur regularly each day. A variety of factors are thought to be the cause of this distress which normally eases up as the baby grows. If attacks are prolonged consult a doctor for advice.

TREATMENT

Make sure the baby's feeding times are relaxed and peaceful. Try to prevent the baby from feeding too quickly as they may take in air with the milk causing flatulence. Make sure that the baby is well 'winded' during and after the feed.
The more peaceful and regular the baby's routine is the greater chance that the colic attacks will gradually subside.
Keep the baby's room at a steady temperature so that the baby neither overheats nor becomes chilly.

APPLICATION

Make up a bottle of Baby Colic Treatment Oil by adding 2 drops of BLEND to 30ml of Sunflower Oil (see Carriers).
If the baby has colic after feeding rub this Treatment Oil sparingly around your baby's tummy. Use very gentle clockwise stroking. This will help to calm the baby. Turn the baby over and repeat the gentle circular movements over the middle of the baby's back.

VAPOURISER

Place a bowl of steaming water in the baby's room, well away from the baby's head. Add 1 drop of BLEND to the water. This allows the molecules of essential oils to evaporate and circulate through the room.
You can also use 1 drop of Dill (anethum graveolens) in the same manner. Dill is used in commercial gripe water.

DIET

If you are breast feeding your baby your own diet is important. Avoid wine, citrus fruits, grapes and fried onions. These have been known to be the cause of the problem.

Baby Coughs and Colds

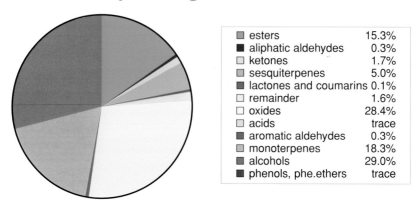

esters	15.3%
aliphatic aldehydes	0.3%
ketones	1.7%
sesquiterpenes	5.0%
lactones and coumarins	0.1%
remainder	1.6%
oxides	28.4%
acids	trace
aromatic aldehydes	0.3%
monoterpenes	18.3%
alcohols	29.0%
phenols, phe.ethers	trace

CCP of BLEND RECIPE

 ◊ *Lavender True* (lavandula angustifolia)

 ◊ *Tea Tree* (melaleuca alternifolia)

 ◊ *Eucalyptus Blue Gum* (eucalyptus globulus)

Lavender True is antiviral, bactericidal and antiseptic. It offers help to treating bronchitis, coughs, sinusitis and TB. Its beautiful familar aroma is soothing and calming.

Tea Tree is strongly antiseptic and bactericidal - excellent for clearing up infections.

Eucalyptus Blue Gum is a decongestant, expectorant, mucolytic. It is used to treat asthma, catarhh, diphtheria, laryngitis, pneumonia, scarlet fever and tonsillitis.

A well balanced chemical blend. Four families take the major share of the oil. The oxides offer help with the congestion of mucous. The esters help to calm the system and the alcohols and monoterpenes can act as tonics.

Chemical constituents to be found in the blend may include:

- linalyl acetate, lavandulyl acetate
- citral
- pinocarvone
- β-caryophyllene, viridiflorene, aromadendrene
- coumarin

- 1.8-cineole
- α-pinene, α-terpinene, γ-terpinene p-cymene, terpinolene
- α-terpineol, terpinen-4-ol, borneol, globulol, lavandulol

BLEND

6 drops	*Lavender True*
6 drops	*Tea Tree*
6 drops	*Eucalyptus*
18 drops	*BLEND*

Make up your *BLEND* using the quantities above - store in a small dark glass bottle fitted with a dropper (see page 20).

TREATMENT

Continuous coughs and cold are distressing both to mother and baby. Some precautions can help to alleviate the frequency of these conditions.
Put 2 drops of *BLEND* into a plant spray full of water. Use this to regularly spray rooms in the home - this will fend off infections. Do not use this spray directly in the baby's room. To help your baby cope with the congestion of the nasal passages place a bowl of warm water under the baby's cot (away from the head end) and add 1 drop of *BLEND* to the water. The vapour carries the molecules around the room and this gently eases the baby's congestion.

TISSUES

If the baby is very stuffed up take a tissue and put 1 drop of *BLEND* on it. Place the tissue safely under the top sheet of the cot.

BATHS

Add 1 drop of *BLEND* to baby's bath water. Swish it round well.

MASSAGE

Make up a bottle of Baby Coughs and Colds Treatment Oil by adding 1 drop of *BLEND* to 15ml of Sunflower Oil (see Carriers).
Massage the baby's chest and back with gentle circular movements.
It is a good idea to do this just before bedtime.
Do not continue the treatments for more than a week at a time.

LIFE STYLE

Provided the baby is well wrapped and protected from cold weather a regular outing in the fresh air will help with the congestion and discomfort that comes with a cold.

▨ esters	56.5%
■ aliphatic aldehydes	1.8%
☐ ketones	2.3%
▨ sesquiterpenes	2.3%
■ lactones and coumarins	trace
☐ remainder	2.3%
☐ oxides	3.7%
☐ acids	trace
▨ aromatic aldehydes	
▨ monoterpenes	26.2%
▨ alcohols	4.9%
■ phenols, phe.ethers	trace

CCP of BLEND RECIPE

    Chamomile Roman (chamaemelum nobile)

    Mandarin (citrus reticulata)

Chamomile Roman is a calming sedative oil. It helps with insomnia and irritabilty. It is highly respected for its calming influence on all systems. It has a fruity apple like aroma. This is a very safe oil most suitable to use with babies and children.

Mandarin is especially good for use with children. It has revitalising properties and helps combat insomnia and anxiety. The fruit was given to the Mandarins as a sign of respect - hence its name. The oil has a sweet sharp floral aroma. It is a member of the rutaceae botanical family which is known to generally aid digestion and skin conditions.

The large proportion of esters in this blend indicates a calming effect will be experienced. Its monoterpenes may well ease digestive problems. The two oils blend well together.

Chemical constituents to be found in the blend may include:

- ▨ angelates, tiglates, butyrates methyl anthranilate
- ■ citral
- ☐ pinocarvone
- ▨ caryophyllene, chamazulene

- ☐ 1.8-cineole
- ▨ α-pinene, γ-terpinene, limonene myrcene, *p*-cymene
- ■ α-terpineol, farnesol, linalool citronellol

BLEND

30 drops	*Chamomile Roman*
10 drops	*Mandarin*
40 drops	*BLEND*

Make up your *BLEND* using the quantities above - store in a small dark glass bottle fitted with a dropper(see page 20).

AILMENT

Fretfulness as a frequent occurrence is very upsetting for everyone. With very young babies it is difficult to decide when the baby has wind, colic, teething pain or a condition that needs medical attention.
If the baby is not hungry or wet check for any other obvious reasons for the baby's discontent. Often loud background noises such as TV or a wrong ambient temperature cause frustration.
Fretful periods tend to decrease if the baby's routine is as peaceful and regular as possible.

FEET

Touch is a wonderful way to ease any anxiety state but you want to avoid continuous cuddling being the only way to comfort your baby. An alternative way is to gently massage the baby's feet. This may sound strange but it is a method handed down from ancient cultures and one adopted by many trained nannies. Make up a bottle of Baby Fretful Treatment Oil by adding 4 drops of *BLEND* to 30ml of Sunflower Oil (see Carriers).

Lay the baby down and rub a little of the Treatment Oil on the baby's feet. Grasp each foot firmly between your thumbs and fingers. Gently massage both feet, simultaneously, by moving your thumbs in a circular rhythmic motion from the centre of the foot to the base of the toes. The baby may well fidget to start with but will usually settle quite quickly and often be comforted to sleep.
You can also use this action to just comfort a baby over his socks or garment without the Treatment Oil.

VAPOURISER

If the baby is fretful at night place a bowl of warm water under the cot but not directly beneath the baby's head. Place 1 drop of *BLEND* in the water. The oil molecules will circulate and have a calming effect.

MASSAGE

A baby enjoys a massage as part of his contact with his parents. Lay the baby in a warm and comfortable position. Using the Treatment Oil gently massage the baby with soft circular strokes. In other words caress your baby and softly sing or talk to them. Spend a little time with the baby lying on his tummy and then a little time on his back. Gently stroke his little limbs.

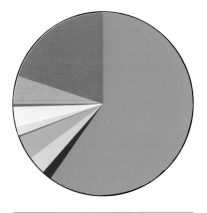

▨ esters	60.0%
■ aliphatic aldehydes	1.5%
☐ ketones	3.5%
▨ sesquiterpenes	4.0%
■ lactones and coumarins	0.1%
☐ remainder	1.9%
☐ oxides	3.5%
☐ acids	trace
■ aromatic aldehydes	0.5%
▨ monoterpenes	4.5%
■ alcohols	20.5%
■ phenols, phe.ethers	trace

CCP of BLEND RECIPE

  Lavender True (lavandula angustifolia)

  Chamomile Roman (chamaemelum nobile)

Lavender True is excellent for the regeneration of skin cells. It heals wounds and scars and is on the whole a calming oil. It is antifugal and bactericidal. It can help with burns, eczema, herpes, psoriasis, spots and wounds.

Chamomile Roman is a member of the compositae botanical family which is known to be generally soothing to the skin and calming to the digestive system. This oil can be used to treat cracked nipples, psoriasis, skin irritations and. surgical scars.

These two oils are particularly suitable for use with young babies. This blend with its large proportion of esters is soothing and calming both to the spirit and to the skin.

Chemical constituents to be found in the blend may include:

- ▨ linalyl acetate, lavandulyl acetate angelates, tiglates, butyrates
- ■ citral
- ☐ pinocarvone, camphor
- ☐ chamazulene, β-caryophyllene
- ▨ coumarin

- ☐ 1.8-cineole
- ■ cuminaldehyde, benzyl aldehyde
- ▨ α-pinene, sabinene
- ■ terpinen-4-ol, α-terpineol, linalool farnesol, lavandulol

BLEND

8 drops	*Lavender True*
8 drops	*Chamomile Roman*
16 drops	*BLEND*

Make up your *BLEND* using the quantities above - store in a small dark glass bottle fitted with a dropper (see page 20).

AILMENT

Most babies suffer from nappy/diaper rash at some time. It is an angry red rash caused by the baby's urine. It is painful and worrying to the baby and needs immediate treatment. Make sure that nappies are never left wet for long. Untreated nappy rash can give rise to fungal infection which causes the skin to become raw and painful. Essential oils are excellent in dealing with this problem.

APPLICATION

Before changing the baby's nappy prepare a bowl of warm water. For each pint of water in the bowl add 1 drop of *BLEND*. Use clean cotton wool pads to gently sponge the baby's bottom.

Make up a pot of Baby Nappy Rash Treatment Ointment by adding 4 drops of *BLEND* to 40ml of Zinc and Castor Oil ointment (see Home Pharmacy).

After washing the baby's bottom make sure it is thoroughly dry and apply the treatment ointment carefully making sure that all areas affected by the rash have been covered.

LIFE STYLE

Change nappies frequently and always give the baby a short time without a nappy on. Air is a natural healer and the baby will enjoy the freedom.

If the nappy rash is severe the skin looks as though it has been burned or scalded. In this case avoid using any plastic protection and use washable pure cotton nappies until the skin heals. When washing the nappies place 6 drops of *BLEND* in the softener used in the rinse cycle of your washing machine or add 2 drops of *BLEND* to rinse water if washing the nappies by hand.

BATHS

Add 1 drop of *BLEND* to the baby's bath.

OTHER OILS

Other oils that are helpful to damaged skin are *Sandalwood* (santalum album) and *Eucalyptus Lemon Scented* (eucalyptus citriodora)

You can substitute these oils for the ones used in the *BLEND* if you wish.

Baby Teething

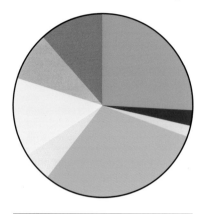

☐ esters	25.7%
■ aliphatic aldehydes	2.3%
☐ ketones	1.7%
☐ sesquiterpenes	31.0%
■ lactones and coumarins	trace
☐ remainder	5.2%
☐ oxides	13.8%
☐ acids	trace
■ aromatic aldehydes	
▨ monoterpenes	8.7%
■ alcohols	11.6%
■ phenols, phe.ethers	trace

CCP of BLEND RECIPE

  Chamomile Roman (chamaemelum nobile)

  Chamomile German (matricaria recutica)

  Ginger (zingiber officinale)

Chamomile Roman is an antiinflammatory, eases pain and is calming to the whole system. It soothes irritability and acts as a general sedative.

Chamomile German is an analgesic bringing relief for the pain. It is recommended in particular for toothache and skin rashes. It also calms the digestive system.

Ginger is an analgesic and temperature reducing. It is good for toothache catarrh, chronic bronchitis and for all side effects of colds. It has a warm pleasant spicy aroma and is to be found in many ancient recipes.

This blend with its large proportion of the ester and sesquiterpene families present offers a calming effect. The oils combine well to treat the pain, lower the temperature and fight any infection.

Chemical constituents to be found in the blend may include:

▨ angelates, ltiglates, butyrates
■ geranial
☐ pinocarvone, gingerone
▨ chamazulene, farnesene, caryophyllene, β-sesquiphellandrene zingiberene, *ar*-curcumene

☐ α-bisabolol oxide, 1.8-cineole
▨ α-pinene, β-pinene, camphene
■ α-bisabolol, α-terpineol, linalool, citronellol, gingerol

BLEND

5 drops	*Chamomile Roman*
5 drops	*Chamomile German*
5 drops	*Ginger*
15 drops	*BLEND*

Make up your *BLEND* using the quantities above - store in a small dark glass bottle fitted with a dropper (see page 20).

AILMENT

By the time a child reaches 2 to 3 years they will have cut their 20 milk teeth. Children vary greatly as to when the teeth arrive. Some babies do not get any teeth until after their first birthday whereas very occasionally a baby is actually born with teeth. The normal pattern is for the first tooth to appear at about 6 months old.

Some babies suffer quite severe symptoms of raised temperature, runny noses and runny stools with a show of considerable discomfort. Other babies seem hardly to notice and their teeth appear with no problems at all.

Disturbed nights result in tiredness and irritation and can set up a vicious circle of upset that is difficult to break. The following treatments will help to break this cycle.

TREATMENT

Make up a bottle of Baby Teething Treatment Oil by adding 2 drops of *BLEND* to 30ml of Sweet Almond Oil (see page 20).

Collect a little of the Treatment Oil onto your fingers and thumb and gently massage the baby's cheek running down the jaw line in soft comforting strokes.

To help ease the soreness of the baby's gums place 1 teaspoonful of the Treatment Oil into a small cup of ice cold water. Take a cotton bud and dip it into the prepared water. Gently wipe the baby's gums with the cotton bud.

Alternatively you can put just one drop of *Chamomile Roman* into a large cup of ice cold water. Swish the water around thoroughly so that the oil mixes well. Now apply to the baby's gum with a cotton bud in the same way as above.

Do not put more than 1 drop of *Roman Chamomile* in the water - if more than 1 drop falls in by accident throw the water away and start again.

FEET

To help the baby settle you can use the foot massage recommended for fretful behaviour.

Grasp each foot firmly between your thumbs and fingers. Gently massage both feet, simultaneously, by moving your thumbs in a circular rhythmic motion from the centre of the foot to the base of the toes. The baby may well fidget to start with but will usually settle quite quickly and often be comforted to sleep. You can do this over the baby's socks or baby suit at any time the baby is restless.

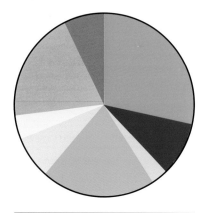

☐ esters	28.5%
■ aliphatic aldehydes	9.4%
☐ ketones	3.5%
☐ sesquiterpenes	20.2%
■ lactones and coumarins	trace
☐ remainder	7.6%
☐ oxides	3.9%
☐ acids	trace
▨ aromatic aldehydes	
☐ monoterpenes	19.8%
▨ alcohols	7.1%
■ phenols, phe.ethers	

CCP of BLEND RECIPE

  💧 *Chamomile Roman* (chamaemelum nobile)

  💧 *Eucalyptus Staigeriana* (eucalyptus staigeriana)

  💧 *Ginger* (zingiber officinale)

Chamomile Roman is potent sedative as well as being a long lasting antiiflammatory. It is highly respected for its calming influence on all systems. It relieves muscular pain and is recommended for back pain, gout and also period pains.

Eucalyptus Staigeriana is a gentle member of the eucalytus family. It has a light lemon aroma in contrast to the harsher camphor aroma of many eucalyptus oils. It is an antiinflammatory recommended for back pain, neck ache and muscle cramps.

Ginger with its warm spicy aroma is recommended for arthritis, back spasms, rhematism and all side effects of colds.

These oils give a well balanced blend of the chemical families.

Chemical constituents to be found in the blend may include:

▨ angelates, tiglates, butyrates menthyl acetate	☐ chamazulene, caryophyllene, zingiberene, β-sesquiphellandrene *ar*-curcumene
■ neral, geranial,citronellal	
☐ pinocarvone, gingerone	▨ α–pinene, limonene
☐ 1.8-cineole	▨ α-terpineol, nerol,citronellol,borneol, linalool, gingerol

BLEND

14 drops	*Chamomile Roman*
14 drops	*Eucalyptus Staigeriana*
14 drops	*Ginger*
42 drops	*BLEND*

Make up your *BLEND* using the quantities above - store in a small dark glass bottle fitted with a dropper (see page 20).

AILMENT

Backache is one of the common chronic conditions that Doctors are asked to deal with. Its possible causes are numerous. Many causes are not serious but occasionally backache can indicate serious problems which need to be identified. The most likely cause is mechanical strain on the back itself. Often the exact reason for the pain is difficult to pin down. Faulty posture or an awkward movement may have stretched ligaments. One common cause of back strain is leaning over at right angles and lifting a heavy weight. Extreme pain may indicate that there is a slipped disc or cracked vertebrae. These severe injuries take several months to heal.

MASSAGE

Back massage with essential oils can be very beneficial to sufferers of chronic back pain. The oils penetrate deeply into muscle tissue and assist the body's natural healing processes. The combination of the oils and gentle body massage bring a good flow of blood to the damaged tissues.

Make up a bottle of Back Pain Treatment Oil by adding 12 drops of *BLEND* to 30ml of Sweet Almond Oil (see page 20). Lie flat on the couch and get a friend to gently massage your back with long flowing strokes with the Treatment Oil. For self treatment you can massage your lower back and around your neck and shoulders. This will still benefit you as the oils are being absorbed into your blood stream.

For chronic sufferers of back pain it is strongly recommended that you book regular appointments with an aromatherapist.

BATHS

Add 8 drops of *BLEND* to your bath.

COMPRESSES

Use hot and cold compresses to alleviate severe pain. Prepare two bowls of water one as warm as you can bear and the other ice cold. Place 4 drops of *BLEND* in each bowl. Soak your compress cloths in each of the bowls. Wring out each cloth and apply alternatively to the painful area. This will increase the flow of blood to the area.

LIFE STYLE

As the major cause of back ache is poor posture, Alexander Technique sessions have an excellent record in helping sufferers. It is highly recommended - try to attend for treatment at least once a week to start with.

——— Blood Pressure High ———

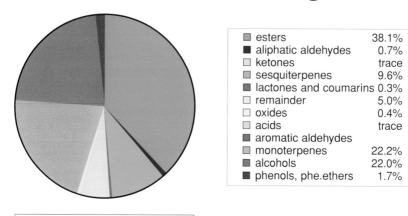

☐ esters	38.1%
■ aliphatic aldehydes	0.7%
☐ ketones	trace
☐ sesquiterpenes	9.6%
■ lactones and coumarins	0.3%
☐ remainder	5.0%
☐ oxides	0.4%
☐ acids	trace
■ aromatic aldehydes	
☐ monoterpenes	22.2%
■ alcohols	22.0%
■ phenols, phe.ethers	1.7%

CCP of BLEND RECIPE

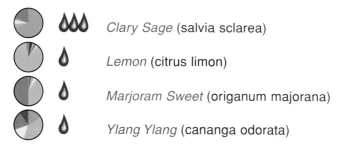

Clary Sage (salvia sclarea)

Lemon (citrus limon)

Marjoram Sweet (origanum majorana)

Ylang Ylang (cananga odorata)

Clary Sage is recommended for high blood pressure and high cholesterol, phlebitis and varicose veins. It is a soothing, calming oil. It has a nutty earthy aroma.

Lemon is a diuretic and helps with obesity, lowers blood pressure and stems bleeding. It is a general rejuvenator due to its oxidising agents.

Marjoram Sweet is a diuretic, vasodilator and balances heart and circulation. It is calming to the nervous system.

Ylang Ylang helps with panic and shock. It slows the heart beat and breathing rate. It has a sweet heavy exotic aroma.

Chemical constituents to be found in the blend may include:

- ☐ linalyl acetate, geranyl acetate terpinyl acetate, benzyl acetate
- ■ citral
- ☐ caryophyllene, germacrene,
- ■ bergaptene
- ☐ α-pinene, β-pinene, γ-terpinene α-terpinene, limonene, myrcene p-cymene, sabinene, ocimene
- ■ sclareol, linalool, terpinen-4-ol, α-terpineol
- ■ methyl eugenol

BLEND

21 drops	*Clary Sage*
7 drops	*Lemon*
7 drops	*Marjoram Sweet*
7 drops	*Ylang Ylang*
42 drops	*BLEND*

Make up your *BLEND* using the quantities above - store in a small dark glass bottle fitted with a dropper (see page 20).

BLOOD PRESSURE

Blood pressure is expressed as the systolic / diastolic readings. A typical reading is 120 / 70. Normal blood pressure is considered to lie between the following range: (100 t0 140) / (60 to 90).

AILMENT

Most cases of high blood pressure have no recognised cause and are known as primary hypertension. Blood pressure that is persistently higher than would be expected should be taken as a warning as it can affect the adequate functioning of the body's organs, for example the kidneys. Some factors, that can be controlled, are often the cause of high blood pressure. For instance - obesity, heavy drinking and smoking. Raised blood pressure definitely shortens life span so it is important to review and correct all possible causes.

BATHS

Add 8 drops of *BLEND* to your bath.

MASSAGE

Make up a bottle of High Blood Pressure Treatment Oil by adding 12 drops of *BLEND* to 30ml of Sweet Almond Oil (see page 20). Get a friend to massage your back with this Treatment Oil. Lie on a couch in a warm room. The massage should be slow, gentle circular movements from the base of the back to the top. A regular visit to an aromatherapist is recommended as it is extremely important to return your blood pressure to its normal level.

LIFE STLYE

Take complete stock of your life style. Cut out smoking and fatty foods. Drink no more than one glass of red wine a day. Attend regular relaxation classes and remove as much stress from your life as possible. Consult the treatments recommended for Anxiety and look at the Appendix for the list of the most stressful happenings in life. Make sure that you have time for leisure and relaxation and that you take regular gentle exercise. Also rest with your feet raised whenever possible.

DIET

Reduce your intake of salt. Follow a low fat diet to ensure that your cholesterol level is kept low.

Supplements
Multi vitamin/mineral tablet
B Complex as per container
Vitamin C 1000mgs twice a day
Garlic capsules as per container
Evening Primrose Oil - 2 tablets daily

Blood Pressure Low

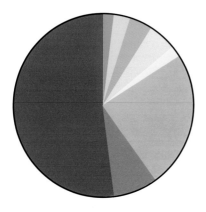

■ esters	1.8%
■ aliphatic aldehydes	trace
□ ketones	3.6%
■ sesquiterpenes	4.0%
■ lactones and coumarins	
□ remainder	4.8%
□ oxides	2.0%
□ acids	trace
■ aromatic aldehydes	trace
■ monoterpenes	24.0%
■ alcohols	7.8%
■ phenols, phe.ethers	52.0%

CCP of BLEND RECIPE

 👁👁 *Clove Bud* (syzygium aromaticum)

 👁 *Pine Scotch* (pinus sylvestris)

 👁👁 *Thyme Red* (thymus vulgaris thymoliferum)

Clove Bud is analgesic, antiviral, bactericidal and stimulating. It is used in many modern pharmaceuticals. Used in traditional medicine for alleviating toothache. It raises blood pressure and regulates the thyroid gland. The oil has a strong spicy aroma.

Pine Scotch is bactericidal, a decongestant and raises blood pressure. It is credited with hormone like behaviour similar to cortisone. It has a fresh forest aroma.

Thyme Red is a strongly stimulating oil. It stimulates the capillaries and raises blood pressure and helps with anaemia. It is a general and neurotonic offering help with depression and stress.
This oil should be avoided during pregnancy.

Chemical constituents to be found in the blend may include:

- ■ bornyl acetate, terpinyl acetate
- □ cryptone, camphor, thujone
- ■ β-caryophyllene
- □ humulene oxide, 1.8-cineole

- □ α-pinene, β-pinene, γ-terpinene limonene, myrcene, sabinene
- ■ terpinen-4-ol, linalool, borneol
- ■ eugenol, aceteugenol, thymol, carvacrol

BLEND

16 drops	*Clove Bud*
8 drops	*Pine Scotch*
16 drops	*Thyme Red*
40 drops	*BLEND*

Make up your *BLEND* using the quantities above - store in a small dark glass bottle fitted with a dropper (see page 20).

BLOOD PRESSURE

Blood pressure is expressed as the systolic / diastolic readings.
A typical reading is 120 / 70. Normal blood pressure is considered to lie between the following range:
(100 to 140) / (60 to 90).

AILMENT

Low blood pressure (hypotension) is not considered as serious as high blood pressure (hypertension) and is rarely a chronic condition. Indeed in this country it is rarely given as a medical diagnosis. However in some countries it is widely identified and probably is used for cases of extreme lassitude with no obvious cause. Low blood pressure can occur after a severe shock causing giddiness and fainting. Another symptom is a feeling of giddiness on standing up quickly - more common amongst the elderly. Certain essential oils help to restore normal blood pressure as they can balance the blood circulation.

BATHS

Add 8 drops of *BLEND* to your bath.

MASSAGE

Make up a bottle of Low Blood Pressure Treatment Oil by adding 12 drops of *BLEND* to 30ml of Sweet Almond Oil (see page 20).
Massage your lower back and the soles of your feet. The Treatment Oil will stimulate the body's immune system and strengthen its resistance. Low blood pressure can occur if the adrenal glands are functioning below par - *Pine Scotch* is recommended for balancing the action of the adrenal glands. *Clove Bud* balances the action of the thyroid gland and *Thyme Red* helps with circulation and stimulates the white corpuscles. This Treatment Oil can also be used to help with ME (Myalgic Encephalomylitis).

LIFE STYLE

Take plenty of regular rest and gentle exercise. Build up your strength gradually, do not rush into extra activities until you are able to cope happily with them.

DIET

Follow a diet of whole foods. Avoid tea, coffee, alcohol and tobacco.

Supplements
Vitamin E 200 I.U.s daily
Vitamin C 1000mgs daily
Iron tablets as per container

Breast Abscess

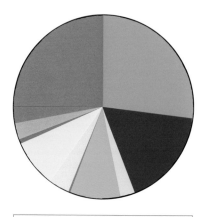

☐ esters	27.6%
■ aliphatic aldehydes	16.6%
☐ ketones	2.4%
☐ sesquiterpenes	10.0%
■ lactones and coumarins	0.2%
☐ remainder	3.6%
☐ oxides	8.4%
☐ acids	
■ aromatic aldehydes	0.6%
☐ monoterpenes	2.6%
■ alcohols	28.0%
■ phenols, phe.ethers	trace

CCP of BLEND RECIPE

  Lavender True (lavandula angustifolia)

  Chamomile German (matricaria recutica)

  Eucalyptus Lemon Scented (eucalyptus citriodora)

Lavender True is excellent for the regeneration of skin cells. It heals wounds and scars and is on the whole a calming oil.

Chamomile German is bactericidal and a decongestant. It helps to lower temperature and assists the skin to heal. It is recommended for various skin disturbances such as psoriasis, rashes, burns, boils, spots and so on.

Eucalyptus Lemon Scented has a fragrant lemon tinged aroma. It has a general calming effect and helps to abate a feverish state. It is used to treat many types of skin damage for example chickenpox sores, wounds and herpes.

Chemical constituents to be found in the blend may include:

☐ linalyl acetate, lavandulyl acetate
   citronellyl acetate
■ citronellal
☐ camphor
☐ caryophyllene, chamazulene
■ coumarin

☐ 1.8-cineole, α-bisabolol oxide
■ cuminaldehyde, benzaldehyde
☐ α-pinene
■ citronellol, α-bisabolol, borneol
   α-terpineol, terpinen-4-ol, lavandulol

15 drops *Lavender True*
 5 drops *Chamomile German*
 5 drops *Eucalyptus Lemon Scented*
25 drops *BLEND*

Make up your *BLEND* using the quantities above - store in a small dark glass bottle fitted with a dropper (see page 20).

AILMENT

Mastitis is inflammation of the breast generally due to nipples becoming sore and damaged. If it does not clear up quickly an abscess can form. An abscess is a collection of pus due to the action of bacterial infection. Essential oils are excellent for helping to fight bacterial infections. If an breast abscess forms during lactation it will be necessary to stop feeding the baby from the infected breast until the infection is cleared. To relieve the pressure, removal of milk from the infected breast can be done gently by hand.

TREATMENT

Apply just 2 drops of neat *Lavender True* to the abscess itself. Next prepare a bowl of warm water and add 5 drops of *BLEND* to it. Make a compress by soaking a clean cotton cloth in the prepared water. Wring the cloth out and wrap gently around the breast. The warmth is comforting. Keep the water warm and repeat this when the breast is giving discomfort. Make up a bottle of Breast Abscess Treatment Oil by adding 12 drops of

BLEND to 30ml of Sweet Almond Oil (see page 20). Apply this Treatment Oil to both breasts, gently massaging them. If you are still feeding from the uninfected breast be sure to wash the nipple thoroughly to remove all the essential oil before feeding the baby. If the abscess does not heal and you have a high temperature consult your doctor. He may decide to prescribe antibiotics - this will mean that breast feeding will have to stop for a while, It can be difficult to re establish it.

LIFE STYLE

To prevent cracked and damaged nipples occurring take advice from your midwife who will assist you to encourage the baby to fasten correctly on the nipple.
After each feed apply the Treatment Oil gently to both breasts and nipples. Always wash the nipples well before feeding the baby.
Geranium leaves can be very soothing and healing if you start to develop sore nipples. Wrap the geranium leaf, furry side to the skin, around your nipple. You can just tuck them inside your bra. They will tingle a little. If, however, you find that they actually irritate the skin stop using them.

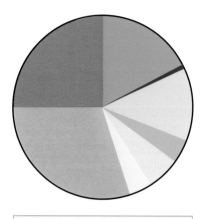

☐ esters	18.7%
■ aliphatic aldehydes	0.5%
☐ ketones	12.0%
☐ sesquiterpenes	3.8%
■ lactones and coumarins	trace
☐ remainder	6.2%
☐ oxides	4.8%
☐ acids	trace
■ aromatic aldehydes	
☐ monoterpenes	29.2%
☐ alcohols	24.8%
■ phenols, phe.ethers	

CCP of BLEND RECIPE

  Eucalyptus Dives (eucalyptus dives)

  Tea Tree (melaleuca alternifolia)

  Chamomile Roman (chamaemelum nobile)

Eucalyptus Dives is an expectorant, decongestant and mucolytic. It is helpful in relieving bronchitis, catarrh and sinusitis. Avoid in pregnancy and with young children. You can substitute it with *eucalyptus staigeriana* for a gentler action.

Tea Tree is strongly bactericidal and is most effective at clearing infections. It is recommended for asthma, bronchitis, catarrh and whooping cough.

Chamomile Roman reduces temperatures and fevers, and generally relaxes the whole body. It is helpful for nervous asthma, irritability, neuralgia and migraines.

Chemical constituents to be found in the blend may include:

- ■ angelates, tiglates, butyrates
- ☐ piperitone, pinocarvone
- ■ β-caryophyllene, chamazulene, aromadendrene, viridiflorene cadinene
- ☐ 1.8-cineole

- ☐ α-pinene, *p*-cymene, limonene α–phellandrene, γ-terpinene α-terpinene, camphene, thujene
- ■ α-terpineol, terpinen-4-ol, linalool globulol, piperitol, viridiflorol, farnesol, *trans*-pinocarveol nerolidol

BLEND

10 drops *Eucalyptus Dives*
20 drops *Tea Tree*
10 drops *Chamomile Roman*
40 drops *BLEND*

Make up your *BLEND* using the quantities above - store in a small dark glass bottle fitted with a dropper (see page 20).

AILMENT

Acute bronchitis is due to the spread of a viral infection from the nose and throat, commonly referred to as a cold settling on the chest. The bronchi are much more vulnerable to infection if they are irritated by smoke or fumes and in some cases even by cold air. A dry uncomfortable cough develops and a fever shows. The inflammation is caused by the over production of mucous in the bronchial tubes. The virus will run its course but essential oils can alleviate the discomfort.

Chronic bronchitis is a much more serious condition accounting for the death of 20,000 people a year in this country. The inflammation of the bronchi becomes very established and the lung tissue receives permanent damage. The efficiency of the lungs becomes impaired and they have difficulty in maintaining the correct levels of oxygen for the body. The major causes of chronic bronchitis are smoking and air pollution.

BATHS

Add 8 drops of *BLEND* to your bath.

TISSUES

Place 3 drops of *BLEND* onto a tissue and inhale deeply. Carry a few prepared tissues in your pocket to use when required.

APPLICATION

Make up a bottle of Bronchitis Treatment Oil by adding 12 drops of *BLEND* to 30ml of Sweet Almond Oil (see page 20).
Rub the Treatment Oil over your chest and back first thing in the morning and last thing at night. The essential oils will enter your blood stream and circulate around the infected lung area helping to clear the congestion and fight the infection.

LIFE STYLE

It is vital not to smoke and to keep away from polluted air. Do not stay in smoke polluted rooms.

DIET

Good foods are vegetables and vegetable soups, pulses, whole grains and all salad foods except for tomatoes. Cut down on dairy foods as they encourage the production of mucous. Avoid bacon, pork and ham. Drink 8 glasses of spring water daily.

Daily Supplements
Multi vitamin/mineral tablet
Vitamin B6 50mgs
Vitamin A 5000 I.U.s
Vitamin C 1000mgs
Six Kelp Tablets

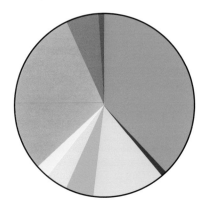

■ esters	38.0%
■ aliphatic aldehydes	1.0%
□ ketones	13.0%
■ sesquiterpenes	5.0%
■ lactones and coumarins	trace
□ remainder	4.0%
□ oxides	2.7%
□ acids	trace
■ aromatic aldehydes	
■ monoterpenes	29.5%
■ alcohols	5.8%
■ phenols, phe.ethers	1.0%

CCP of BLEND RECIPE

  Hyssop (hyssopus officinalis)

  Juniper Berry (juniperus communis)

  Chamomile Roman (chamaemelum nobile)

Hyssop is antiinflammatory, antiseptic and a sedative. It helps bruises, dissolves boils and swellings and is recommended for rheumatism. This oil should be avoided in cases of epilepsy and also should not be used during pregnancy. .

Juniper Berry is a diuretic and is particularly useful in clearing fluid retention. It is recommended for cellulite, obesity, oedema, painful joints, psoriasis and stiffness. This oil is a powerful detoxifying agent. It helps to eliminate uric acid from the system. Avoid during pregnancy and do not use if kidneys are inflamed.

Chamomile Roman is recommended for gout. It will also exert a soothing influence on the whole system.

Chemical constituents to be found in the blend may include:

- ■ bornyl acetate, methyl myrtenate angelates, tiglates, butyrates
- □ pinocamphone, isopinocamphone pinocarvone, camphor
- ■ caryophyllene, cadinene, humulenes chamazulene, germacrene
- ■ umbelliferone
- □ 1.8-cineole, caryophyllene oxide
- ■ α-pinene, β-pinene, γ-terpinene sabinene, limonene, myrcene camphene, *p*-cymene, thujene
- ■ α-terpineol, terpinen-4-ol, borneol linalool, *trans*-pinocarveol, geraniol
- ■ methyl chavicol(estragole)

BLEND

10 drops	*Hyssop*
10 drops	*Juniper Berry*
20 drops	*Chamomile Roman*
40 drops	*BLEND*

Make up your *BLEND* using the quantities above - store in a small dark glass bottle fitted with a dropper (see page 20).

AILMENT

Bursitis is literally inflammation of the bursa. A bursa is a small sac filled with fluid that lubricates the joints by allowing skin, muscles and tendons to move smoothly over the bones. The inflammation can be bactericidal or due to conditions such as rheumatism. It is nearly always caused by repeated pressure, friction or injury. Names for bursitis attacks such as 'housemaid's knee', 'tennis elbow', 'dustman's shoulder' etc. are still in common use.
In bursitis extra fluid collects around the joint impeding movement and causing heat, swelling and pain. Arthritis and gout can also give rise to bursitis.

APPLICATION

To reduce the heat and swelling prepare an ice cold bowl of water and add 5 drops of *BLEND*. Use a cotton cloth to make a compress. Soak the cloth in the prepared water, wring out and apply to the inflamed area. Another way to cool the area is to freeze a cardboard cup of water - the ice will protrude above the lip of the cup. You can massage this gently over the swollen area.

MASSAGE

Make up a bottle of Bursitis Treatment Oil by adding 12 drops of *BLEND* to 30ml of Sweet Almond Oil (see page 20).
Rub the Treatment Oil gently around the affected area at least twice daily. The oils will penetrate the skin and help to combat the infection. *Juniper Berry* is a diuretic which will help to reduce the swelling.

BATHS

Add 8 drops of *BLEND* to your bath. Take plenty of time to soak in the bath. The warmth will comfort the pain and the oils will help the infection.

LIFE STYLE

Once the swelling begins to subside you can exercise the affected joint daily. Exercise for only a minute or two at a time to start with. Repeat this frequently during the day. Avoid any pressure on the joint and avoid any repetitive use of it.

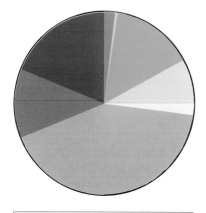

■ esters	2.1%
■ aliphatic aldehydes	
□ ketones	0.5%
■ sesquiterpenes	14.8%
■ lactones and coumarins	trace
□ remainder	8.0%
□ oxides	1.8%
□ acids	trace
■ aromatic aldehydes	
■ monoterpenes	42.0%
■ alcohols	12.1%
■ phenols, phe.ethers	18.7%

CCP of BLEND RECIPE

  Juniper Berry (juniperus communis)

  Cypress (cupressus sempervirens)

  Patchouli (pogostemon cablin)

 Oreganum (origanum vulgaris)

Juniper Berry is recommended for breaking down cellulite and removing excess body fluid Avoid in pregnancy and if kidneys are inflamed.

Cypress regulates, balances and is a good decongestant. Recommended for cellulite, and rheumatism. Constricts blood vessels and combats excesses.

Patchouli is an astringent, decongestant and an excellent oil for encouraging good skin condition.

Oreganum a powerful oil that is a diuretic and cleanses the body by causing sweating. Avoid in pregnancy.

Chemical constituents to be found in the blend may include:

- ■ linalyl acetate, terpinyl acetate
- □ patchoulenone, isopatchoulenone
- ■ caryophyllene, cadinene, cedrene patchoulenes, humulenes, α-guaiene
- □ 1.8-cineole, manoyl oxide, guaiene-oxide, bulnesene oxide, caryophyllene oxide

- ■ α-pinene, β-pinene, γ-terpinene α-terpinene, limonene, sabinene p-cymene, myrcene
- ■ α-terpineol, sabinol, pogostol patchouli alcohols, manool, linalool, cedrol, guaiol, bulnesol
- ■ carvacrol, thymol

BLEND

10 drops	*Juniper Berry*
10 drops	*Cypress*
10 drops	*Patchouli*
10 drops	*Oreganum*
40 drops	*BLEND*

Make up your *BLEND* using the quantities above - store in a small dark glass bottle fitted with a dropper (see page 20).

AILMENT

Research in France, Italy and Germany has revealed that constipation, poor lymphatic system, poor circulation and weak functioning of the kidney and liver are more common in women prone to cellulite. Cellulite shows as lumpy puckered tissue giving the skin an appearance similar to orange peel. It tends to collect on the thighs and buttocks and sometimes on the arms as well. Essential oils can help to break down these fatty deposits and attention to diet will also be beneficial.

MASSAGE

Make up a bottle of Cellulite Treatment Oil by adding 12 drops of *BLEND* to 30ml of Sweet Almond Oil (see page 20).
Massage the Treatment Oil twice daily all around the affected body areas. Use a firm pressure and work in strong circular movements using the palm of your hand. Increase the pressure as you become accustomed to the massage action.
To improve your blood and lymph circulation organise to have regular professional massage treatments.

BATHS

Add 8 drops of *BLEND* to your bath. Soak well and allow plenty of time for the oils to be absorbed into the body. They will begin to break down the fatty tissues.

SKIN BRUSHING

Skin brushing will help stimulate the lymph system. Use a long handled natural- bristle hair brush or a friction glove. Friction gloves can be purchased from the chemist. Follow a daily routine - brush the complete body, except for the face, first thing in the morning and last thing at night. Start gently and increase the pressure as the body becomes used to the treatment.

DIET

Some naturopaths recommend a diet of 75% raw food to prevent the cellulite from forming and to eliminate the existing cells.

Other recommended foods are :
Beetroot juice - good for liver function
Celery - good for excess fluid
Cucumber - good for kidneys
Watermelon - good for excess fluid

General weight loss usually improves the condition considerably.

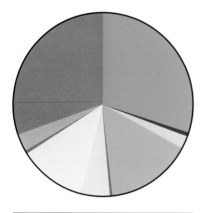

esters	30.0%
aliphatic aldehydes	0.7%
ketones	2.7%
sesquiterpenes	15.0%
lactones and coumarins	0.2%
remainder	4.1%
oxides	13.0%
acids	
aromatic aldehydes	0.7%
monoterpenes	3.0%
alcohols	30.6%
phenols, phe.ethers	trace

CCP of BLEND RECIPE

  Lavender True (lavandula angustifolia)

  Chamomile German (matricaria recutica)

Lavender True is excellent for the regeneration of skin cells. It heals wounds and scars and is on the whole a calming oil. It also has analgesic properties and helps with anxiety and migraines. It is recommended for burns, eczema, psoriasis, spots and blisters.

Chamomile German is analgesic, antiinflammatory, temperature reducing and hormone like. It is useful for treating acne, boils, burns, insect bites, psoriasis, rheumatism, toothache, wounds and ulcers. This oil is a cooling treatment for the skin. The deep blue colour is due to the chamazulene which forms during distillation.

This blend of two oils will give relief to the itchiness of the patient's skin whilst guarding against infection getting into the chickenpox spots.

Chemical constituents to be found in the blend may include:

- linalyl acetate, lavandulyl acetate geranyl acetate
- citral
- octanone, camphor
- β-caryophyllene, farnesene chamazulene
- coumarin, umbelliferone
- en-yn-dicycloether, *cis*-spiro-ether

- 1.8-cineole, α-bisabolol oxide linalool oxide, caryophyllene oxide
- cuminaldehyde, benzaldehyde
- ocimene, camphene, limonene
- terpinen-4-ol, α–terpineol, borneol α-bisabolol, linalool, lavandulol geraniol

BLEND

28 drops *Lavender True*
14 drops *Chamomile German*
42 drops *BLEND*

Make up your *BLEND* using the quantities above - store in a small dark glass bottle fitted with a dropper (see page 20).

AILMENT

A most infectious and common virus. An attack of the chickenpox virus (varicella) often confers lifelong immunity although the virus always remains in the body and can break out again. Because of this immunity it is mainly suffered in childhood. The virus takes about 14 days to incubate and the sufferer is highly infectious 4 days before the rash appears until the final scabs have healed. The rash starts, together with a temperature, as small raised spots which progress into very unsightly inflamed blisters. The spots start on the trunk and spread to the face and limbs. Despite the horrendous appearance of the skin with such ugly blisters the skin usually makes a complete recovery, especially if the patient resists the urge to scratch.

If contracted as an adult the attack is likely to be much more severe and the patient can feel very ill for the first few days.

The same virus is responsible for both shingles and herpes.

An outbreak of shingles can result in ongoing pain for some months. Medical treatment for shingles should be sought - especially if the infection gets into the eyes.

TREATMENT

Make up a bottle of Chickenpox Treatment Lotion by adding 20 drops of *BLEND* to 100ml of Calamine Lotion.

Apply the Treatment Lotion all over the body twice a day. Rest in bed whilst the fever lasts and get as much sleep as possible.

BATHS

Add 4 drops of *Lavender True* and 1 cup of bicarbonate of soda to your bath. This will help to relieve the itching.

VAPOURISER

Place 4 drops of *Tea Tree* (melaleuca alternifolia) in a plant spray full of water. Spray the rooms in the house as a help to combat the spread of the infection.

DIET

Drink raw vegetable and fruit juices, lemon and orange juice in particular. Lemon tea is also refreshing and beneficial.

☐ esters	1.7%
■ aliphatic aldehydes	trace
☐ ketones	17.2%
☐ sesquiterpenes	27.6%
■ lactones and coumarins	trace
☐ remainder	2.2%
☐ oxides	20.8%
☐ acids	trace
■ aromatic aldehydes	
■ monoterpenes	4.0%
■ alcohols	26.5%
■ phenols, phe.ethers	

CCP of BLEND RECIPE

  Cedarwood Atlas (cedrus atlantica)

  Eucalyptus Blue Gum (eucalyptus globulus)

  Mint Peppermint (mentha piperita)

Cedarwood Atlas clears mucous and is recommended for bronchitis. It belongs to the Pinaceae family which is generally known for aiding respiratory conditions and is highly antiseptic.

Eucalyptus Blue Gum clears nasal passages, reduces temperature and is excellent for all colds.

Mint Peppermint lowers fever, is a good expectorant and generally helps mental fatigue.

The blend is well balanced. The ketones and oxides help with the congestion. The alcohols make it highly antiseptic. The sesquiterpenes are calming.

Chemical constituents to be found in the blend may include:

☐ atlantone, pinocarvone, menthone
☐ cadinene, aromadendrene, germacrene, caryophyllene

☐ 1.8-cineole
■ atlantol, cedrol, globulol, pinocarveol, menthol

BLEND

20 drops *Cedarwood Atlas*
10 drops *Eucalyptus Blue Gum*
10 drops *Mint Peppermint*
40 drops *BLEND*

Make up your *BLEND* using the quantities above - store in a small dark glass bottle fitted with a dropper (see page 20).

GARGLE

A *Teatree* oil gargle is helpful at the onset of all colds especially if a sore throat is a symptom.
Add 1 drop of *Teatree* (melaleuca alternifolia) oil to a glass of warm boiled water.
Gargle at frequent intervals.

MASSAGE

Add 12 drops of the *BLEND* to 30ml of Sweet Almond Oil to make up a supply of Common Cold Treatment Oil (see page 20).
Alternatively add 12 drops of the *BLEND* to 30ml of body cream or lotion
Massage chest, neck and upper back areas morning and night.
Concentrate thumb massage around the vertebrae as this stimulates the action of the oils.
A facial massage with this Treatment Oil helps sinusitis sufferers.
Rub a small amount of Treatment Oil under the nostrils when going to bed.

ROOM SPRAY

Add 12 drops of the *BLEND* to 1 litre of water. Spray freely in any room.

TISSUES

Place 2 to 4 drops of the *BLEND* onto a paper tissue.
Wrap the tissue in foil and pop it in your pocket so that you can inhale the vapours from the tissue at regular intervals during the day.
To ease congestion at night place such a tissue on the soles of your feet. The vapour from the oils passes around the body as you sleep.

VAPOURISER

Place 4 to 6 drops of the *BLEND* in the vapouriser.
It helps to keep the vapouriser going in any room where you are spending any length of time.
This also guards against others contracting your condition.

BATHS

Place 8 drops of the *BLEND* into a warm bath.
Relax and inhale the vapours.
This is particularly helpful before going to bed.

DIET

Two or three garlic tablets each day are recommended.
Cut down on all dairy food as this encourages the production of mucous in the system.
Take regular doses of vitamin C tablets or drinks.
Follow a light healthy diet of fruit and vegetables.

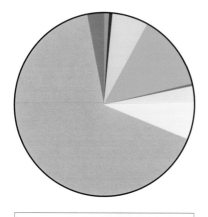

☐ esters	1.0%
■ aliphatic aldehydes	0.8%
☐ ketones	6.6%
☐ sesquiterpenes	12.8%
■ lactones and coumarins	0.2%
☐ remainder	3.3%
☐ oxides	6.2%
☐ acids	trace
▨ aromatic aldehydes	trace
▨ monoterpenes	66.0%
▨ alcohols	3.1%
■ phenols, phe.ethers	trace

CCP of BLEND RECIPE

  Orange Bitter (citrus aurantium amara)

  Black Pepper (piper nigrum)

  Rosemary (rosmarinus officinalis)

Orange Bitter is a calming cheering oil that is generally helpful to the digestive system. It treats both nervous indigestion and constipation. Also it is a stimulant to the liver.

Black Pepper is a warming and stimulating oil. It is extremely helpful to the digestive system, stimulating the liver and pancreas. It is recommended for constipation, flatulence and indigestion and also tones the colon muscles.

Rosemary is an antispasmodic and analgesic and stimulates bile production. Traditionally the Greeks and Romans considered it to be a sacred plant bringing peace and comfort. It is a smooth muscle relaxant. Do not use if epilepsy is suspected.

Chemical constituents to be found in the blend may include:

- ▨ linalyl acetate, geranyl acetate, citronellyl acetate, bornyl acetate
- ■ undecanal, citral
- ☐ piperitone, dihydrocarvone camphor, carvone, thujone
- ▨ β-caryophyllene, bisabolene humulenes, farnesene, copaene
- ☐ caryophyllene oxide, 1.8-cineole
- ▨ piperonal
- ▨ limonene, α-pinene, myrcene β-pinene, sabinene, camphene, *p*-cymene, phellandrene, ocimene
- ▨ linalool, nerol, α-terpineol, citronellol terpinen-4-ol, borneol

BLEND

16 drops	*Orange Bitter*
16 drops	*Black Pepper*
8 drops	*Rosemary*
40 drops	*BLEND*

Make up your *BLEND* using the quantities above - store in a small dark glass bottle fitted with a dropper (see page 20).

AILMENT

Constipation, strictly speaking, is a symptom rather than an ailment. It is an indication that for some reason the body is not able to function as it should. Life style, diet and each person's constitution affect bowel habits. It is quite normal for some people to have 3 bowel actions a day and quite normal for other people to have a bowel movement just 3 times a week. Irregular and frequent small hard motions are the signs of constipation problems looming.

MASSAGE

Make up a bottle of Constipation Treatment Oil by adding 12 drops of *BLEND* to 30ml of Sweet Almond Oil (see page 20).
Rub the oil all over the abdomen. Cover the whole area starting at the hair line and working up to the chest. Use gentle circular strokes.
You can gently rub a little of the Treatment Oil around and just inside the anus the encourage the intestinal reflex to work.

LIFE STYLE

A readily identifiable cause of constipation is the taking of drugs. Morphine and its derivatives such as codeine are almost certain to have constipation as a side effect. Some drugs for lowering blood pressure and some anti-depressants are equally guilty.
Failure of the intestinal reflexes as a result of old age is common and chronic. It then becomes necessary to take gentle laxatives to deal with the problem. However in general do not resort to purges or strong laxatives as they can set up a vicious circle of events.
Take regular exercise to condition your stomach and back muscles this can in turn aid the bowel movements. Visit the lavatory at regular intervals - take a good book and relax allowing the body to resume its regular habits.

DIET

Drink at least 8 glasses of mineral water a day. Good natural laxatives are broccoli, cabbage, prunes and figs. Bran is also recommended and in general stick to a diet that includes plenty of fluid and fibre.

Cramp

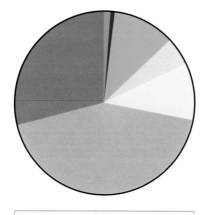

▨	esters	1.1%
■	aliphatic aldehydes	0.7%
☐	ketones	
▨	sesquiterpenes	11.3%
■	lactones and coumarins	trace
☐	remainder	5.1%
☐	oxides	10.0%
☐	acids	
■	aromatic aldehydes	
▨	monoterpenes	43.1%
▨	alcohols	28.7%
■	phenols, phe.ethers	trace

CCP of BLEND RECIPE

 🌢🌢🌢 *Marjoram Sweet* (origanum majorana)

 🌢🌢 *Mandarin* (citrus reticulata)

 🌢🌢 *Chamomile German* (matricaria recutica)

Majoram Sweet is analgesic, antispasmodic, balancing and calming. It helps circulation and is vasodilatory. Used for treating muscle aches, bruising, cramps and rheumatism. Known in folk lore as 'joy of the mountain'.

Mandarin is antispasmodic and revitalising offering help for anxiety and stress. Balances metabolic rate. This fruit was given to the Madarins as a mark of respect.

Chamomile German is again an antispasmodic oil. It calms the system down and helps with back pain and any muscular spasms. Good for intestinal colic and flatulence.

Chemical constituents to be found in the blend may include:

- ▨ linalyl acetate, terpinyl acetate, geranyl acetate, methyl anthranilate
- ■ citral, citronellal
- ▨ caryophyllene, cadinene chamazulene, farnesene
- ☐ en-yn-dicycloether, *cis*-spiro ether
- ☐ α–bisabolol oxide
- ▨ β-pinene, α-terpinene, γ–terpinene, *p*-cymene, myrcene, limonene, ocimene, sabinene
- ▨ linalool, borneol, α-terpineol, terpinen-4-ol, α-bisabolol
- ■ carvacrol, eugenol, thymol

BLEND

18 drops *Majoram Sweet*
12 drops *Mandarin*
12 drops *Chamomile German*
42 drops *BLEND*

Make up your *BLEND* using the quantities above - store in a small dark glass bottle fitted with a dropper (see page 20).

AILMENT

Cramp is a painful spasm of a muscle - very often suffered in a calf or thigh muscle. The muscles contract involuntarily and suddenly causing severe pain. The contraction can last for several minutes. Even the bravest of people cry out at such pain. The known causes for these muscle contractions to be triggered involuntarily are a shortage of salts in the system, due maybe to excessive sweating, or bodily fatigue or a deficient blood supply due to poor circulation.

FIRST AID

To relieve the cramp it is necessary to stretch the cramped muscles.
If the thigh muscles are cramped sit down, straighten out the leg and get a helper to lift the foot in one hand whilst pushing firmly down on the knee with the other hand.
Another possible way to break the contraction is to press firmly on the nail of the big toe and apply strong pressure to both the front and the back of the toe.
For hand cramp force the fingers apart and place the finger tips firmly down on a cold surface.

MASSAGE

Make up a bottle of Cramp Treatment Oil by adding 12 drops of *BLEND* to 30ml of Sweet Almond Oil (see page 20).
Massage gently around the muscle area as soon as the cramp has subsided.
Before going to bed at night massage the whole leg upwards with the Treatment Oil.
Also massage the Treatment Oil well into your feet. It is most important that your feet are warm and that the blood is circulating to them. Put warm bed socks on and place a soft pillow beneath your feet. In this way your feet will remain warm throughout the night.

BATHS

Add 8 drops of *BLEND* to your bath.

DIET

If the cause of your cramp attacks is poor circulation follow a low fat diet to ensure that your cholesterol level is kept low.
If the cause is due to lack of salts in the blood then increase your intake of salt for a while to restore the balance.

Supplements
Multi vitamin/mineral tablet
B Complex as per container
Vitamin C 1000mgs a day
Garlic capsules as per container
Evening Primrose Oil - 2 tablets daily.

Cystitis

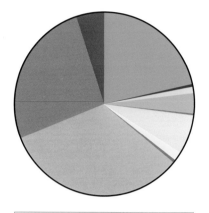

☒ esters	20.6%
■ aliphatic aldehydes	0.4%
☐ ketones	1.6%
☒ sesquiterpenes	4.2%
■ lactones and coumarins	0.1%
☐ remainder	7.1%
☐ oxides	1.6%
☐ acids	trace
▨ aromatic aldehydes	0.4%
☒ monoterpenes	32.6%
▨ alcohols	26.4%
■ phenols, phe.ethers	5.0%

CCP of BLEND RECIPE

  Basil Sweet European (ocimum basilicum)

  Lavender True (lavandula angustifolia)

 Pine Scotch (pinus sylvestris)

Basil Sweet European is antiviral, bactericidal. It is a stimulant and tonic having a strong cleansing effect on the body. It cleanses the kidneys, helps with congested prostate and attacks cistitis.

Lavender True is a calming gentle oil and is strongly bactericidal. It not only clears infections it also helps sore and damaged skin to heal quickly.

Pine Scotch is antiinflammatory antiseptic. It has a hormone like action and brings the body back to balance. It has a fresh forest like aroma. It is acknowledged that pine forests produce a healing environment due to evaporation of the essential oil from the pine needles.

Chemical constituents to be found in the blend may include:

- ☒ linalyl acetate, fenchyl acetate, methyl cinnamate, lavandulyl acetate bornyl acetate, terpinyl acetate
- ■ citronellal, citral
- ☐ octanone, camphor, cryptone
- ☒ β-caryophyllene, cadinene, copaene, guaiene, farnesene
- ■ coumarin, umbelliferone
- ☐ 1.8-cineole, linalool oxide
- ▨ cuminaldehyde, benzaldehyde
- ☒ *cis*-ocimene,α-pinene, β-pinene, limonene ,myrcene, sabinene
- ▨ α-terpineol, linalool, borneol, lavandulol, terpinen-4-ol
- ■ eugenol, methyl chavicol

BLEND

8 drops	*Basil Sweet European*
16 drops	*Lavender True*
16 drops	*Pine Scotch*
40 drops	*BLEND*

Make up your *BLEND* using the quantities above - store in a small dark glass bottle fitted with a dropper (see page 20).

AILMENT

Cystitis causes a burning pain on passing urine and urges frequent trips to the lavatory to find it is only possible to pass a few drops. Also the sufferer can fell quite unwell in themselves.
Cystitis is an inflamed membrane in the bowel usually caused by bacterial infection that has travelled up the urinary passage. Due to the fact that this passage is much shorter in women than in men women are the main sufferers of this condition. It can also be triggered by food allergy, chemical sensitivity, bruising during intercourse and vaginal thrush.
It can clear up within hours or may develop into a life long problem.
If blood appears in the urine seek medical advice.

TREATMENT

Make up a bottle of Cystitis Treatment Oil by adding 12 drops of *BLEND* to 30ml of Sweet Almond Oil (see page 20).
Use this soothing Treatment Oil and apply to gently to the entrance to the urinal passage. Do this 2 or 3 times a day

Once a day lie quietly and massage this Treatment Oil over the abdomen, hips and lower back.
Help your body combat the infection by taking plenty of rest if necessary take some bed rest.

BATHS

Add 8 drops of *BLEND* to your bath. Take 2 or 3 baths a day soak for at least 10 to 15 minutes. This will help you to deal with the discomfort.

DIET

Drink at least 8 glasses of spring water a day.
Until the condition clears avoid, as far as possible, all acid producing foods such as:-
citrus or sour fruits,
vinegars,
animal proteins such as eggs, fish, meat and cheese.

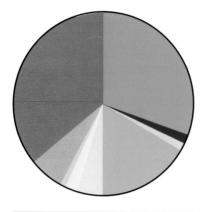

▨ esters	30.4%
■ aliphatic aldehydes	1.8%
☐ ketones	1.6%
▨ sesquiterpenes	16.2%
■ lactones and coumarins	trace
☐ remainder	4.7%
☐ oxides	2.3%
☐ acids	1.0%
▨ aromatic aldehydes	
▨ monoterpenes	6.0%
▨ alcohols	36.0%
■ phenols, phe.ethers	trace

CCP of BLEND RECIPE

  Ginger (zingiber officinale)

  Sandalwood (santalum album)

  Chamomile Roman (chamaemelum nobile)

Ginger is antispasmodic and temperature reducing. Its warm spicy aroma is comforting. Excellent oil for all digestive upsets. Used in many ancient recipes.

Sandalwood has a musty lingering aroma that creates a feeling of peace. It is a sedative and calming oil.

Chamomile Roman helpful for intestinal colic. It is antispasmodic, calming and sedative and also reduces temperature and fever. This oil is highly respected for its calming influence on all systems. Known as the plant's physician as it protects neighbouring plants from infections.

Chemical constituents to be found in the blend may include:

- ▨ angelates, tiglates, butyrates, propionates
- ■ geranial, citronellals
- ☐ gingerone, santalone, pinocarvone
- ▨ β-sesquiphellandrene, zingiberene santalenes, curcumenes, farnesene chamazulene, caryophyllene
- ☐ 1.8-cineole
- ☐ nortricycloekasantalic acid
- ▨ α-pinene, β-pinene, camphene, limonene, phellandrene, sabinene
- ■ citronellol, linalool, borneol, gingerol santalols, tricycloekasantalol, farnesol, nerolidol, α-terpineol, *trans*-pinocarveol

BLEND

8 drops	*Ginger*
16 drops	*Sandalwood*
16 drops	*Chamomile Roman*
40 drops	*BLEND*

Make up your *BLEND* using the quantities above - store in a small dark glass bottle fitted with a dropper (see page 20).

AILMENT

Most diarrhoea is due to inflammation of the intestines. This inflammation is commonly caused by viruses, bacterial food poisoning or less commonly by larger parasites such as amoebic dysentery or worms. Nervous upset can also cause the condition as disturbances of the endocrine hormonal output can over activate the intestinal action.
Irritable colon, a common complaint, is often the result of anxiety and sometimes made worse by constant taking of laxatives. Laxatives can irritate the colon and cause it to form too much mucous which is then mistaken for diarrhoea.
If the diarrhoea persists without relief for 2 to 3 days seek medical advice.

PREVENTION

Always make sure that food is thoroughly washed and clean.Take extra precautions if travelling and only drink bottled water.
Establish a regular pattern of eating wholesome foods and try to establish a regular bowel action. Try to reduce stress levels (see Appendix).

MASSAGE

Make up a bottle of Diarrhoea Treatment Oil by adding 12 drops of *BLEND* to 30ml of Sweet Almond Oil (see page 20).
Massage your abdomen and lower back. Work with gentle circular stokes in a clockwise direction. Repeat the treatment every 2 to 3 hours whilst the condition persists. Take time to relax and unwind.

BATHS

Add 8 drops of *BLEND* to your bath. Take time to relax and the essential oils will help to balance your system.

DIET

It is very important not to become dehydrated during an attack of diarrhoea. The body looses salts faster than it can replace them. Make a replacement drink by preparing a glass of warm water to which you add some sugar and a pinch of salt. Take frequent small drinks of this. It is also possible to buy sachets of prepared minerals from the chemist if you prefer.
Another drink that often settles an upset stomach is a glass of warm water with one teaspoon of honey and one drop of *Mint Peppermint* (mentha piperita) Again sip it gradually.
Avoid all foods that are likely to create acid levels as these will prompt the intestine to produce too much mucous.
It is a good idea to fast for several hours and then gradually introduce bland foods. This helps the system to recover.

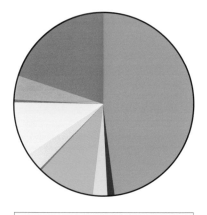

▨ esters	48.0%
■ aliphatic aldehydes	1.2%
☐ ketones	2.8%
▨ sesquiterpenes	10.2%
■ lactones and coumarins	0.1%
☐ remainder	3.3%
☐ oxides	9.8%
☐ acids	trace
■ aromatic aldehydes	0.4%
▨ monoterpenes	3.8%
■ alcohols	20.4%
■ phenols, phe.ethers	trace

CCP of BLEND RECIPE

  Chamomile Roman (chamaemelum nobile)

  Lavender True (lavandula angustifolia)

 Chamomile German (matricaria recutica)

Chamomile Roman has a very cooling effect on the skin and calms all the body systems down. It is excellent for easing the irritation caused by eczema.

Lavender True helps to heal skin wounds and keeps infection at bay. Its beautiful aroma is also very soothing.

Chamomile German is good for all states of tension and nervous reaction to stress. This oil is recommended for acne, allergies, boils, burns, psoriasis, rashes, ulcers and wounds. It has a warm herby aroma.

Chemical constituents to be found in the blend may include:

- ▨ angelates, tiglates, linalyl acetate, geranyl acetate, lavandulyl acetate
- ■ citral
- ☐ pinocarvone, octanone, camphor
- ☐ chamazulene, β–caryophyllene farnesene
- ■ coumarin, umbelliferone

- ☐ en-yn-dicycloether, *cis*-spiro-ether
- ☐ α–bisabolol oxide. 1.8-cineole, caryophyllene oxide, linalool oxide
- ▧ cuminaldehyde, benzaldehyde
- ■ α-bisabolol, farnesol, nerolidol, α-terpineol, trans-pinocarveol terpinen-4-ol, linalool, borneol, geraniol, lavandulol

BLEND

16 drops	*Chamomile Roman*
16 drops	*Lavender True*
8 drops	*Chamomile German*
40 drops	*BLEND*

Make up your *BLEND* using the quantities above - store in a small dark glass bottle fitted with a dropper (see page 20).

AILMENT

Eczema appears as an inflamed area of skin which is extremely itchy. It often develops into blisters that weep and form crusty scabs.

There are two types of eczema. The first called contact eczema appears within minutes of contact with substances that cause the skin to react. The substances can be as diverse as gold and wax polish. The second type of eczema called atopic eczema is much more difficult to deal with. In this case the cause is difficult to track down. Very often people prone to these inexplicable attacks of eczema are allergy sufferers. It is also believed that extreme unhappiness or life stress can prompt outbreaks of eczema. Eczema in young children tends to gradually diminish as they grow up.

Unfortunately for adult atopic eczema sufferers it can take a long time to discover the cause.

APPLICATION

Make up a bottle of Eczema Treatment Oil by adding 12 drops of *BLEND* to 30ml of Sweet Almond Oil (see page 20).

To help with the discomfort apply the Treatment Oil to the affected areas night and morning.

If the irritation is very bad during the day make up a pot of eczema Treatment Lotion by adding 12 drops of *BLEND* to 30ml of lotion. Apply the lotion gently to the area.

Try to overcome the urge to scratch at all times as it will only irritate the skin further. Just placing your hand firmly over the irritating area may help you to cope.

BATHS

Add 8 drops of *BLEND* to your bath. Make sure the water temperature is not too hot. Taking a bath can really help to cope with the irritation.

LIFE STYLE

If you suspect the eczema attack may be linked to personal stress and emotional upset you must try to resolve your situation. Consult the list of stressful situations listed in the Appendix. It may be advisable to seek some professional counselling. A useful address for eczema sufferers is:

National Eczema Society, Tavistock House, Tavistock Square, London, WC1.

DIET

If you suspect that your eczema attack is due to food allergy then devise a method for tracking down the guilty party. Start by restricting your diet to just a few items. If that is successful just add an extra item at a time. Professional consultants can help you set up such a programme.

Emotional Stress

▨ esters	30.0%
■ aliphatic aldehydes	1.6%
☐ ketones	1.4%
▨ sesquiterpenes	9.1%
■ lactones and coumarins	3.0%
☐ remainder	4.8%
☐ oxides	0.4%
☐ acids	trace
■ aromatic aldehydes	
▨ monoterpenes	20.3%
■ alcohols	27.4%
■ phenols, phe.ethers	2.0%

CCP of BLEND RECIPE

  Geranium (pelargonium graveolens)

  Bergamot (citrus bergamia)

  Ylang Ylang (cananga odorata)

Geranium is an excellent all round balancer, eliminates waste and congestion. It calms nervous fatigue and regulates hormonal function.

Bergamot calms anxiety. It also assists skin to heal. It can be most helpful at combating depression. It encourages confidence and revitalises.

Ylang Ylang helps with anxiety, fear, depression and panic. It slows the breathing pace. It has a sweet heavy exotic aroma.

The largest chemical families in this blend are the esters, sesquiterpenes, monoterpenes and alcohols. Thus the blend shows a good balance between calming and cheering aspects.

Chemical constituents to be found in the blend may include:

- ▨ linalyl acetate, citronellyl acetate benzyl acetate, geranyl acetate
- ■ citral
- ☐ menthone
- ▨ β-caryophyllene, germacrene β-bisabolene, guaiazulene

- ■ bergaptene
- ☐ *cis*-rose oxide
- ▨ α-pinene, β-pinene, γ-terpinene limonene, α-terpinene
- ■ linalool, farnesol, geraniol citronellol
- ■ eugenol, safrole

BLEND

8 drops	*Geranium*
24 drops	*Bergamot*
8 drops	*Ylang Ylang*
40 drops	*BLEND*

Make up your *BLEND* using the quantities above - store in a small dark glass bottle fitted with a dropper (see page 20).

MASSAGE

Make up a bottle of Emotional Stress Treatment Oil by adding 12 drops of *BLEND* to 30ml of Sweet Almond Oil (see page 20).
Take time to sit quietly and massage your feet and hands with this Treatment Oil.
If possible ask a friend or partner to give you a soothing shoulder massage. A great deal of tension is held in the shoulders and neck. Emotional stress is a condition that is greatly helped by visiting a professional aromatherapist at regular intervals. Weekly visits to start with can prove extremely helpful.

RELAXATION

It is vital to find time to relax. Make time during the day to sit quietly in peaceful surroundings.
Taking tuition in the Alexander Technique can be beneficial. Many people with demanding work find this helpful.

ANXIETY ATTACKS

Many people suffering from emotional stress are liable to panic attacks. For immediate relief put 3 drops of *Bergamot* oil onto a tissue and inhale gently. If you are prone to such attacks carry a tissue with you.

LIFE STYLE

Take gentle walks, attend relaxation sessions such as Alexander Technique and Yoga. Daily swimming is also excellent for helping the body relax. Consult the list of most stressful life situations in the Appendix.

DIET

Follow a light healthy diet of fruit and vegetables. Cut out any heavy fatty foods.
Avoid strong stimulants such as coffee and tea.

OTHER ESSENTIAL OILS

Other oils that can be helpful during times of emotional stress are:

Palma Rosa, Lavender True, Juniper Berry, Sweet Majoram, Rose and Sandalwood

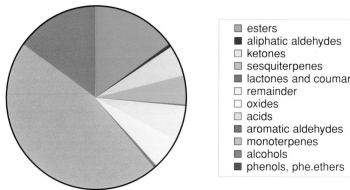

▢ esters	15.2%
■ aliphatic aldehydes	0.3%
▢ ketones	5.5%
▢ sesquiterpenes	5.2%
■ lactones and coumarins	0.1%
▢ remainder	6.4%
▢ oxides	5.7%
▢ acids	trace
■ aromatic aldehydes	0.3%
▨ monoterpenes	46.3%
■ alcohols	15.0%
■ phenols, phe.ethers	trace

CCP of BLEND RECIPE

 🌢🌢🌢 *Juniper Berry* (juniperus communis)

 🌢🌢 *Lavender True* (lavandula angustifolia)

 🌢 *Rosemary* (rosmarinus officinalis)

Juniper Berry is excellent for cleansing the body. It is recommended for cellulite, fluid retention, obesity, clearing fluid from oedemas and eliminating uric acid from painful joints.

Lavender True is antiinflammatory and antiseptic. It is excellent for helping skin conditions and is a generally balancing oil.

Rosemary is a stimulating oil. It is a diuretic and a decongestant. It stimulates the memory and helps with fatigue and depression.

Chemical constituents to be found in the blend may include:

- ▨ linalyl acetate, geranyl acetate, lavandulyl acetate, fenchyl acetate bornyl acetate, terpinyl acetate
- ■ citral
- ▢ camphor, carvone, thujone, octanone
- ▢ β-caryophyllene, cadinene, humulenes, germacrene
- ▨ coumarin, umbelliferone
- ▢ 1.8-cineole, linalool oxide, caryophyllene oxide
- ▨ cuminaldehyde, benzaldehyde
- ▨ α-pinene, γ-terpinene, myrcene, limonene, sabinene, *p*-cymene camphene, ocimene, thujene
- ▨ terpinen-4-ol, α-terpineol linalool, borneol, geraniol, lavandulol

BLEND

21 drops *Juniper Berry*
14 drops *Lavender True*
 7 drops *Rosemary*
42 drops *BLEND*

Make up your *BLEND* using the quantities above - store in a small dark glass bottle fitted with a dropper (see page 20).

AILMENT

Fluid retention, known medically as oedema, is the build up of water in the body's fluid tissue to an abnormal level. The body is 60% water which means that an average body has 40 litres of water to be distributed. For this average body to be healthy it needs 3 litres of this water in its blood, 25 litres of this water in its cells and 12 litres of this water in the fluid that the cells are immersed in, called the body's fluid tissue.
Water passes out of the blood in the capillaries into the body's fluid tissue as the pressure from the heart pumping reaches it.
Water passes from the body's fluid tissue back into the blood in the capillaries drawn back by the level of protein in the blood.
Water passes from the blood in the capillaries to the body's tissue fluid drawn out by the level of salt in the body's tissue fluid.
Thus if the pressure from the heart beat is not correct or the level of protein in the blood is not correct or the level of salt in the body tissue fluid is not correct the distribution of the water in the body becomes unbalanced. The amount of water in the body's fluid tissue becomes too much and a swelling results.

If the capillaries become damaged through such things as injury, surgery, burning etc they can no longer control the balance of this water flow and the tissue swells as the excess is unable to pass back into the blood stream.

TREATMENT

If the cause of the fluid retention is due the fact that there is too much salt in the body tissue this can be helped by diuretic action. Juniper Berry and Rosemary will help in this case. Fluid retention occurs if you stand for long periods or remain sitting on long journeys. This because the veins are working against gravity and pressure builds on the capillaries. This will right itself when you can move naturally.

MASSAGE

Make up a bottle of Fluid Retention Treatment Oil by adding 12 drops of *BLEND* to 30ml of Sweet Almond Oil (see page 20).
Massage back of legs, lower back and abdomen. The endocrine glands also affect the balance of the water held in the body tissue. This can cause fluid retention to occur during menstruation. Start to use this massage 2 to 3 days before a period.

DIET

Reducing salt in your diet may be helpful if the retention is caused by too much salt in the system.
Fluid retention in the body tissue is not closely linked to the amount of fluid you drink so cutting this down is not a solution.

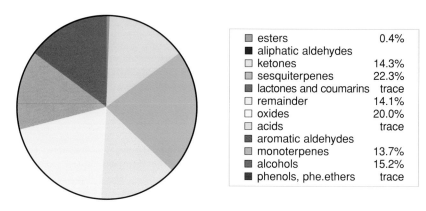

■ esters	0.4%
■ aliphatic aldehydes	
□ ketones	14.3%
■ sesquiterpenes	22.3%
■ lactones and coumarins	trace
□ remainder	14.1%
□ oxides	20.0%
□ acids	trace
■ aromatic aldehydes	
■ monoterpenes	13.7%
■ alcohols	15.2%
■ phenols, phe.ethers	trace

CCP of BLEND RECIPE

  Tagetes (tagetes glandulifera)

  Carrot Seed (daucus carota)

 Chamomile German (matricaria recutica)

Tagetes is antifungal, antiinflammatory, antiseptic and helps skin infections to clear. It is recommended for athlete's foot, bunions, callouses, corns. It has a strong marigold aroma. The tagetes plant is often planted in the vegetable garden to keep pests at bay.

Carrot Seed acts in a hormonal way regulating body functions. It is recognised as an antiageing agent and is used to treat chilblains, gout and skin wounds.

Chamomile German is a generally soothing oil that has a calming effect on all nervous tensions. It is particular useful in tackling allergic skin reactions.

Chemical constituents to be found in the blend may include:

- ■ geranyl acetate
- ■ citral
- □ tagetone, tagetenones, carvone
- ■ daucene, bisabolene, elemene, caryophyllene, chamazulene, farnesene
- □ en-yn-dicycloether, cis-spiro-ether
- □ α-bisabolol oxide
- □ valeric acid
- ■ salicylaldehyde
- ▨ limonene, α-pinene, β-pinene myrcene, camphene
- ■ α-bisabolol, linalool
- ■ asarone

BLEND

12 drops	*Tagetes*
6 drops	*Carrot seed*
24 drops	*Chamomile German*
42 drops	*BLEND*

Make up your *BLEND* using the quantities above - store in a small dark glass bottle fitted with a dropper (see page 20).

FOOT CARE

Our feet are incredibly important to our general well being. The natural massage of the sole of the feet during walking stimulates all the pressure points and the muscle action in the legs keeps our circulation level up.
Healthy well cared for feet can be the basis of a happy life.

GENERAL CARE

Make up a bottle of Foot Care Treatment Oil by adding 4 drops of *BLEND* to 30ml of Sweet Almond Oil (see page 20).
Whenever possible use a little of this Treatment Oil and treat your feet to a relaxing massage with it. Better still get a friend to do it for you. You will find this extraordinarily beneficial.

FOOT BATH

After a tiring day prepare a warm foot bath by putting 4 drops of *BLEND* in the bowl of water. Relax and soak your feet well.

BLISTERS

As soon as a blister appears put 1 drop of *Lavender True* and 1 drop of *Tea Tree* directly onto it. If the blister has not burst this will cause the fluid to clear, if it has already burst the oils will heal the wound and protect it from infection.

CORNS

Make up a bottle of Corn Treatment Oil by adding 1 drops of *Tagetes* to 30ml of Sweet Almond Oil. Use this to massage your feet from time to time - it will help to prevent corns from forming.

BUNIONS

Massage around the bunion with the Foot Care Treatment Oil 3 times daily.

LIFE STYLE

Always cherish your feet. Make sure that all your footwear fits well and is comfortable to walk in. Spend some time walking around barefooted.
If your feet have problems such as ingrowing toe nails or painful corns visit a qualified chiropodist and get expert advice and treatment.

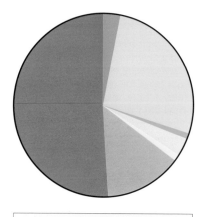

■ esters	3.2%
■ aliphatic aldehydes	trace
□ ketones	26.8%
■ sesquiterpenes	1.2%
■ lactones and coumarins	trace
□ remainder	3.3%
□ oxides	0.9%
□ acids	trace
■ aromatic aldehydes	
■ monoterpenes	13.8%
■ alcohols	50.8%
■ phenols, phe.ethers	trace

CCP of BLEND RECIPE

 ▲▲▲ *Coriander* (coriandrum sativum)

 ▲▲ *Mint Spearmint* (mentha spicata)

Coriander is a tonic to the digestive system. It is analgesic, antispasmodic, hormone like and will help with mental fatigue and sadness. For the digestive system it will help with anorexia, colic, bad breath, enteritis and indigestion. The aroma is sweet spicy and woody. The herb has been used since ancient times as a herb of happiness - it is used in Benedictine and Chartreuse liqueurs.

Mint Spearmint is a digestive tonic and is recommended for bile flow, dyspepsia, flatulence, liver, vomiting. The aroma is spicy warm and minty. Avoid in pregnancy and do not use with young children.

Valued highly as a culinary herb. The water from distillation is used to relieve coughs, colic, hiccoughs and flatulence.

Chemical constituents to be found in the blend may include:

- ■ cis-carvyl acetate, linalyl acetate
- ■ decyl aldehyde
- □ camphor, carvone, menthone
- ■ elemene, farnesene, bourbonene caryophyllene
- ■ umbelliferone, bergaptene
- □ 1.8-cineole

- ■ α-pinene, α-terpinene, γ-terpinene limonene, β-pinene phellandrene, camphene
- ■ linalool, α-terpineol, geraniol, menthol, borneol
- ■ anethole

BLEND

24 drops *Coriander*
16 drops *Mint Spearmint*
40 drops *BLEND*

Make up your *BLEND* using the quantities above - store in a small dark glass bottle fitted with a dropper (see page 20).

AILMENT

When gas collects in the intestines it can inflict a great deal of discomfort. The flatulence can be caused by swallowing air by eating too quickly. Also if you are tensed up the digestive system can be affected in this way. Further flatulence can build up in the lower part of the intestine due to the fermentation of food. Sometimes the pressure builds up to such an extent that the swelling can push up into the rib cage. In such a case shortness of breath can be experienced and also angina like pains.
Less commonly, flatulence can be the result of gall stones or the gall bladder being under par.
Should your digestion become really troublesome and also accompanied by weight loss then seek medical advice.

BATHS

Add 8 drops of *BLEND* to your bath. Allow plenty of time to soak and let the tension relax.

MASSAGE

Make up a bottle of Gastric Flatulence Treatment Oil by adding 12 drops of *BLEND* to 30ml of Sweet Almond Oil (see page 20).
Massage the whole of the abdomen to ease the discomfort. Use gentle circular strokes.

VAPOURISER

Place 5 drops of *BLEND* in your vapouriser and let the molecules circulate in the room.

LIFE STYLE

Organise if possible for meal times to be peaceful. Eat slowly. Avoid belching as that also traps air in the stomach.

DIET

Foods that are likely to cause flatulence are the starchy cellulose foods such as wheat, peas, onions and potatoes etc.

DRINKS

Prepare a glass of warm water with a teaspoon of honey and 1 drop of *Mint Peppermint* (mentha piperita). Sip slowly.

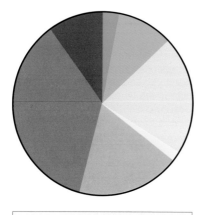

☐ esters	3.0%
■ aliphatic aldehydes	
☐ ketones	
☐ sesquiterpenes	10.0%
■ lactones and coumarins	
☐ remainder	20.6%
☐ oxides	1.6%
☐ acids	trace
■ aromatic aldehydes	
☐ monoterpenes	19.2%
☐ alcohols	35.6%
■ phenols, phe.ethers	10.0%

CCP of BLEND RECIPE

  Basil Sweet European (ocimum basilicum)

  Carrot Seed (daucus carota)

Basil Sweet European is antifungal, antiseptic, antiviral and bactericidal. It helps with allergies, gout, acne and reduces the uric acid in the system. The aroma is clear, spicy and sweet. This oil is used extensively in Ayurvedic medicine.

Carrot Seed is antiageing, a decongestant. It has a balancing effect on the body and helps to regulate the functions. It dilates blood vessels and is an immune stimulant. It is a diuretic and recommended for gout.
This oil has a dry sweet aroma. It is excellent for general health and well being. Widely used in food flavouring

Chemical constituents to be found in the blend may include:

☐ linalyl acetate, fenchyl acetate, methyl cinnamate, geranyl acetate

☐ β-caryophyllene, daucene, elemene, bisabolene

☐ 1.8-cineole

☐ α-pinene, β-pinene, γ-terpinene, limonene, *cis*-ocimene, *p*-cymene, camphene

☐ terpinen-4-ol, α–terpineol, linalool, citronellol, geraniol, carotol, daucol

■ methyl chavicol, eugenol, asarone methyl eugenol

BLEND

16 drops *Basil Sweet European*
24 drops *Carrot Seed*
40 drops *BLEND*

Make up your *BLEND* using the quantities above - store in a small dark glass bottle fitted with a dropper (see page 20).

AILMENT

Gout is the build up of uric acid that forms crystals around the joints. Although all foods are a potential source of uric acid they are not normally the main culprit. The body synthesis should maintain the correct levels of uric acid in the tissues, however over synthesis can result in the uric acid crystals being deposited. Thus this ailment is likely to be due to hereditary biochemical problems.
Attacks of gout appear without warning - a single joint is suddenly inflamed and extremely painful. The uric acid crystals are seen by the body as 'foreign bodies'.
Unfortunately the immune system attacks and in a sense attacks the body itself. Grumbling arthritis is also a form of gout.
It can become a dangerous condition if the uric acid crystals form in the kidneys.

BATHS

Put 8 drops of *BLEND* in your bath water. Soak well, the warmth eases the pain.

MASSAGE

Make up a bottle of Gout Treatment Oil by adding 12 drops of *BLEND* to 30ml of Sweet Almond Oil (see page 20).
Massage the Treatment Oil near to the inflamed joint but not actually on it. Get a friend to give you a back massage as this will allow the oils to enter the blood stream and travel to the affected area.

COMPRESSES

Prepare a bowl of warm water add 4 drops of *BLEND*. Use a cotton cloth to make a compress. Soak the cloth in the prepared water, wring out and wrap around the affected joint.

FOOT BATHS

If the feet are affected treat them to frequent foot baths. Prepare a bowl of warm water and add 4 drops of *BLEND*. Soak the feet well in the prepared water.

DIET

Foods high in uric acid are liver and kidneys.
Cut back on red meats, dairy produce and alcohol. Concentrate on fish and green vegetables.

Daily Supplements
Vitamin C 1000mgs
Vitamin E 250mgs
One teaspoon of Codliver Oil plus 5 drops of Evening Primrose Oil.

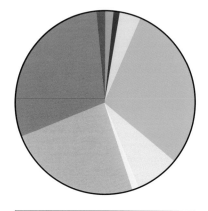

esters	1.6%
aliphatic aldehydes	1.1%
ketones	3.6%
sesquiterpenes	29.1%
lactones and coumarins	
remainder	8.5%
oxides	1.1%
acids	trace
aromatic aldehydes	trace
monoterpenes	23.6%
alcohols	29.8%
phenols, phe.ethers	1.6%

CCP of BLEND RECIPE

Patchouli (pogostemon cablin)

Myrrh (commiphora myrrha)

Cypress (cupressus sempervirens)

Patchouli is antiviral, astringent, bactericidal, decongestant and a tonic to the immune system. It is recommended for phlebitis and varicose veins. It heals damaged tissue. The aroma is sweet and earthy.

Myrrh is antiinflammatory, antifungal, antiseptic and astringent. It is excellent for helping skin tissue repair.

Cypress is astringent, contracts the blood vessels and is a decongestant. It is recommended for broken capillaries, haemorrhoids, rheumatism and sweaty feet.

Chemical constituents to be found in the blend may include:

- myrrholic ester,α-terpinyl acetate
- 2-butanal
- patchoulenone, isopatchoulenone methyl isobutyl ketone, curzerenone
- α-guaiene, patchoulenes, elemene, cedrene, cadinene, α-bulnesene, seychellenes, caryophyllene, copaene
- guaiene oxide, bulnesene oxide caryophyllene oxide, 1.8-cineole

- myrrholic acid
- cinnamaldehyde, cuminaldehyde
- α-pinene, β-pinene, Δ3-carene , p-cymene, camphene, limonene dipentene,
- guaiol, bulnesol, pogostol, cedrol patchouli alcohols, myrrh alcohols α–terpineol, borneol, sabinol
- eugenol

BLEND

6 drops   *Patchouli*
27 drops   *Myrrh*
15 drops   *Cypress*
48 drops   *BLEND*

Make up your *BLEND* using the quantities above - store in a small dark glass bottle fitted with a dropper (see page 20).

AILMENT

Haemorrhoids are distended veins in the rectum about one inch above the anus. Lack of dietary fibre leading to constipation may be the cause of them forming. Once the pain and discomfort of haemorrhoids is present that also sets up constipation so there is a vicious circle to break. Another cause of haemorrhoids is the pressure on the veins by a pregnant uterus. Thus haemorrhoids are a common occurrence during pregnancy. Any compression of the veins can cause haemorrhoids. Fortunately although a nuisance, haemorrhoids usually heal up given careful attention. However it is advisable to get a medical diagnosis to confirm that the bleeding is due to haemorrhoids. The early stages of cancer have very similar symptoms so its well worth checking up.

BATHS

Add 8 drops of *BLEND* to your bath. Take frequent baths soaking and relaxing in them is very beneficial. If you have a sitz bath this is ideal.

APPLICATION

Add 12 drops of *BLEND* to 30ml of KY jelly. Rub this all around the anal area. Repeat this 2 or 3 times a day.

LIFE STYLE

Take time to rest regularly to relieve the pressure on the veins. Always rest with your feet raised. In pregnancy take regular 10 minute rests throughout the day. This is very beneficial and will keep your energy levels up.

SUPPOSITORIES

Chemists can supply you with suppositories which can be extremely helpful with the discomfort experienced with haemorrhoids.

DIET

Try to avoid getting constipated. Follow a wholefood diet with a good level of fibre.

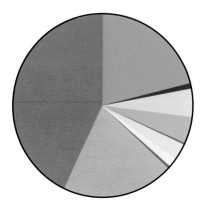

■ esters	21.6%
■ aliphatic aldehydes	0.9%
□ ketones	5.1%
■ sesquiterpenes	4.2%
■ lactones and coumarins	0.1%
□ remainder	2.9%
□ oxides	1.7%
□ acids	trace
■ aromatic aldehydes	0.4%
■ monoterpenes	20.2%
■ alcohols	42.9%
■ phenols, phe.ethers	trace

CCP of BLEND RECIPE

Lavender True (lavandula angustifolia)

Marjoram Sweet (origanum majorana)

Mint Peppermint (mentha piperita)

Lavender True is analgesic, antispamodic, balancing and calming. It lowers blood pressure and is recommended for anxiety, headaches, insomnia and migraines.

Marjoram Sweet, known as 'joy of the mountain' is analgesic, antispamodic, balancing and helps with depression and headaches. It is recommended for clearing obsessional thought patterns.

Mint Peppermint acts as a local anaesthetic and is helpful to mental fatigue, nervous exhaustion migraines and stress.

Chemical constituents to be found in the blend may include:

■ linalyl acetate, terpinyl acetate, geranyl acetate, menthyl acetate lavandulyl acetate

■ citral

□ menthone, isomenthone, pulegone octanone, camphor

□ germacrene, β-caryophyllene

■ aesculetine, menthofuran, coumarin

□ 1.8-cineole, caryophyllene oxide

■ cuminaldehyde, benzaldehyde

■ β-pinene, α-terpinene, γ-terpinene, p-cymene, myrcene, limonene, ocimene, sabinene, α-pinene

■ terpinen-4-ol, α-terpineol, linalool, borneol, geraniol, lavandulol menthol, neomenthol

■ carvacrol, eugenol

BLEND

20 drops *Lavender True*
20 drops *Majoram Sweet*
 5 drops *Mint Peppermint*
45 drops *BLEND*

Make up your *BLEND* using the quantities above - store in a small dark glass bottle fitted with a dropper (see page 20).

AILMENT

Everybody experiences headaches. Unfortunately it is almost impossible to be sure of the causes. It can be part of any illness from a small boil to high blood pressure. The meninges that cover the brain are the tissues that perceive the pain as the brain itself is fairly insensitive. If something irritates the meninges this irritation is likely to manifest itself as a headache. For some chronic headache sufferers it proves very difficult to pinpoint the causes. Migraine, the most extreme form of headaches, is equally difficult to tie down to a single cause. All that can be said is that a headache is triggered by the blood vessels in the head. An exception to this is sinusitis where the pain is related to the bone of the skull.

However despite the difficulty in tracking down the many causes of headaches by far the most common cause is over tiredness and anxiety. In these states the muscles of the neck and shoulders tense up and the pressure results in a headache. Severe and sudden headpain or headaches that persist long term should be reported to your doctor to check that no serious condition is causing pressure to build up.

MASSAGE

Make up a bottle of Headache Treatment Oil by adding 12 drops of *BLEND* to 30ml of Sweet Almond Oil (see page 20).
Headaches that start at the back of the head are almost certain to be caused by muscle tension. Get a friend to massage your neck. Gentle strokes down the back of the neck, firmer pressure around the shoulders and kneading action on the tight muscle band each side of the neck.

TISSUES

Place 2 drops of *BLEND* on a tissue and inhale at frequent intervals. Pop prepared tissues in your pocket.

BATHS

Put 8 drops of *BLEND* in your bath. Soak and relax.

APPLICATION

Place 2 drops of *Lavender True* on your fingers and rub gently around your temples. Also rub your fingers across the back of your neck. Try to lie down away from the light and close your eyes for a rest period. Pinching the bridge of your nose may also help.
Hot and cold compresses may also lessen the pain by stimulating the circulation.

DIET

Avoid chocolate, cheese and red wine if you suffer from migraine.

Herpes Simplex

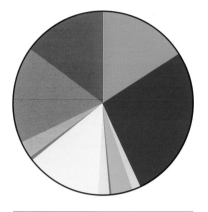

■	esters	16.2%
■	aliphatic aldehydes	27.0%
□	ketones	1.5%
■	sesquiterpenes	3.3%
■	lactones and coumarins	0.1%
□	remainder	2.7%
□	oxides	13.8%
□	acids	trace
■	aromatic aldehydes	0.3%
▦	monoterpenes	3.0%
■	alcohols	17.0%
■	phenols, phe.ethers	15.1%

CCP of BLEND RECIPE

  Eucalyptus Blue Gum (eucalyptus globulus)

  Eucalyptus Lemon Scented (eucalyptus citriodora)

  Clove Bud (syzygium aromaticum)

 Lavender True (lavandula angustifolia)

Eucalyptus Blue Gum is antiseptic and decongestant. Recommended for chicken pox, herpes simplex and measles.

Eucalyptus Lemon Scented is antiviral, bactericidal and used to treat scabs, sores, herpes simplex and chicken pox.

Clove Bud is a powerful oil used to clear skin problems such as infected acne and herpes simplex blisters.

Lavender True excellent for helping damaged skin to heal.

Chemical constituents to be found in the blend may include:

■ linalyl acetate, geranyl acetate, lavandulyl acetate, citronellyl butyrate, α-terpinyl acetate citronellyl citronellate
■ citronellal, citral
□ menthone, pinocarvone, camphor
□ β-caryophyllene, humulenes aromadendrene

■ coumarin, umbelliferone
□ 1.8-cineole, caryophyllene oxide
■ cuminaldehyde, benzaldehyde
▦ α-pinene, limonene, *p*-cymene,
▦ citronellol, terpinen-4-ol, α-terpineol, borneol, linalool, lavandulol
■ eugenol, isoeugenol, aceteugenol

BLEND

7 drops   *Eucalyptus Globulus*
14 drops *Eucalyptus Lemon Scented*
7 drops   *Clove Bud*
14 drops *Lavender True*
42 drops *BLEND*

Make up your *BLEND* using the quantities above - store in a small dark glass bottle fitted with a dropper (see page 20).

AILMENT

Herpes simplex is a virus that once in the body lies dormant in a nerve ganglion. It can erupt at any time. There are 2 different strains of this virus.
Herpes Simplex Type I is the well known cold sore. Almost everybody is infected with this virus having come into contact with it as a child. The eruptions can appear anywhere but most commonly they appear on the face near the mouth. The virus erupts when the body system is depleted due to some other infection. This is why cold sores so often appear during a cold. They are tiresome but harmless. However they can become dangerous if contracted by a baby prone to allergic eczema and also if they break out near the eyes. In either of these cases seek medical advice.
Herpes Simplex Type II causes similar lesions but it attacks the sexual organs and is called genital herpes. It is much more common now and is registered as a sexually transmitted disease. The initial attack of genital herpes is quite distressing. The sufferer will feel ill and the attack will take 10 days or so to run its

course. Subsequent attacks are not so severe.
Herpes zoster is the chicken pox and shingles virus. In the case of shingles it is advisable to seek medical advice as once again it become very dangerous if it attacks the eyes. There is no known cure for this virus.

TREATMENT

Keep the lesions clean and dry. As the virus can be transferred to the eyes keep your fingers away from your eyes. Use clean flannels and towels every day.

APPLICATION

Make up a bottle of Herpes Simplex Treatment Oil by adding 12 drops of *BLEND* to 30ml of Sweet Almond Oil and 5 drops of Calendula Oil. (see page 20).
To ease the discomfort gentle apply the Treatment Oil, using cotton wool pads, to the affected parts 2 or 3 times daily.

BATHS

To ease the discomfort from genital herpes put 8 drops of *BLEND* in your bath. Soak and relax twice a day.

DIET

Try to build up your immune system so that the body is not prone to attacks of the herpes virus.

Daily Supplements
Multi vitamin/mineral tablet
Vitamin C1000mgs

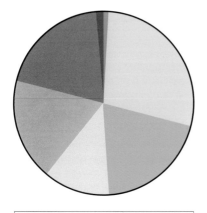

▨ esters	trace
■ aliphatic aldehydes	1.0%
□ ketones	28.0%
▨ sesquiterpenes	19.5%
■ lactones and coumarins	trace
□ remainder	12.5%
□ oxides	
□ acids	trace
■ aromatic aldehydes	trace
▨ monoterpenes	17.5%
■ alcohols	20.0%
■ phenols, phe.ethers	1.5%

CCP of BLEND RECIPE

  🝆 *Tagetes* (tagetes glandulifera)

  🝆 *Myrrh* (commiphora myrhha)

Tagetes is antiseptic, antifungal, bactericidal, antiinflammatory and helps to generate new cell growth to repair damaged skin. It is recommended for many skin related problems such as corns, calluses, infected sores. The aroma is a strong pungent marigold - the plants are known to deter pests and are often planted to protect other plants from damage.

Myrrh is well know to help serious skin conditions such as ulcers, gangrene and bed sores. It is antiviral, antiseptic, antiinflammatory. The oil has a drying effect which helps healing to occur. The aroma is musky and smoky.

This blend produces a very earthy aroma.

Chemical constituents to be found in the blend may include:

- ▨ myrrholic ester
- ■ citral, 2-butanal
- □ tagetone, tagetenones, carvone
  methyl isobutyl ketone, curzerenone
- ▨ elemene, heerabolene, cadinene,
  copaene, curzerene, lindestrene
- □ myrrholic acid

- ▨ cinnamaldehyde, cuminaldehyde
  salicylaldehyde
- ▨ pinenes, limonene, ocimene,
  myrcene, camphene, limonene
- ■ linalool, myrrh alcohols
- ■ eugenol

BLEND

16 drops *Tagetes*
16 drops *Myrrh*
32 drops *BLEND*

Make up your *BLEND* using the quantities above - store in a small dark glass bottle fitted with a dropper (see page 20).

AILMENT

Impetigo is a highly contagious bacterial infection of the skin. Outbreaks at schools occur from time to time and if not checked quickly a minor epidemic can occur. The sores are particularly unsightly and will persist for a long time if not treated properly. Although a child will not feel ill they remain highly infectious. The staphylococci actually form small clusters of abscesses which show up as red spots with yellow crusts. They usually affect sufferer's face, hands or knees.

TREATMENT

As soon as the condition is recognised it is important to start careful treatment. If not attended to the infection will spread to other parts of the skin making the healing process more difficult.
First of all attend to the infected pus to keep the area as clean as possible. Prepare a bowl of cool boiled water and add 5 drops of *Lavender True* (lavandula angustifolia). Using cotton wool pads gentle wash the pus from the sores. Use fresh cotton wool each time so that the water remains clean from infection.

With a fresh bowl of water again with 5 drops of *Lavender True* prepare a compress using a clean cotton cloth. Soak the cloth in the water and then gently lay it on the sores. Hold in place for a few minutes.

COMPRESSES

For a compress that will be left in place prepare a large bowl of just boiled water. Cut a piece of lint that is double the size of the area you wish to treat. Put 2 drops of *BLEND* in the water and soak the lint then wring it out. Fold the lint in half and place in position. Either bandage it or if necessary use plaster tape to secure it.
Leave the lint in position for 2 to 3 hours then leave the sore open to the air.
It will take time and patience to encourage the sores to heal but essential oils are exceptionally helpful.
Make sure that the sufferer is unlikely to pass the infection on. If necessary they should stay at home for a few days.

BATHS

Put 4 drops of *BLEND* in baths.

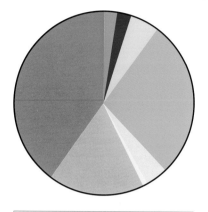

☐ esters	2.5%
■ aliphatic aldehydes	2.5%
☐ ketones	5.0%
☐ sesquiterpenes	27.5%
■ lactones and coumarins	trace
☐ remainder	4.3%
☐ oxides	0.7%
☐ acids	trace
▨ aromatic aldehydes	
▨ monoterpenes	17.5%
▨ alcohols	40.0%
■ phenols, phe.ethers	trace

CCP of BLEND RECIPE

  Coriander (coriandrum sativum)

  Ginger (zingiber officinale)

Coriander has a sweet spicy woody aroma. It has been used since ancient times - considered the herb of happiness. It is a tonic to the digestive system and helps with colic, bad breath, anorexia, enteritis and indigestion. It belongs to the Umbelliferae botanical family which is known to aid digestion.

Ginger has a warm pleasant spicy aroma and is a very comforting oil. It is useful for helping hangovers, indigestion, flatulence, nausea and seasickness. It is an analgesic, antispasmodic and prevents stomach griping. It is used in many ancient remedies. The oil is distilled from unpeeled dried ground rhizome.

Chemical constituents to be found in the blend may include:

- ▨ geranyl acetate, linalyl acetate
- ■ decyl aldehyde, geranial, citronellal
- ☐ camphor, carvone, gingerone
- ▨ β-sesquiphellandrene, zingiberene, *ar*-curcumene
- ■ umbelliferone, bergaptene

- ☐ 1.8-cineole
- ▨ γ-terpinene, *p*-cymene, α–pinene, limonene, β-pinene, camphene,
- ▨ linalool, α-terpineol, geraniol, citronellol, borneol, gingerol
- ■ anethole

BLEND

20 drops *Coriander*
20 drops *Ginger*
40 drops *BLEND*

Make up your *BLEND* using the quantities above - store in a small dark glass bottle fitted with a dropper (see page 20).

AILMENT

For indigestion due to flatulence consult the notes on Gastric Flatulence.
Indigestion may take the form of the regurgitation of acid, or partly digested food, from the stomach into the oesophagus. This results in the pain commonly described as heart burn and another term to describe the indigestion is 'acid stomach'. This reaction from the stomach can be caused by overeating, constricted clothing, obesity and physical exercise immediately after eating. However regular attacks can also be caused by a loose muscle in the oesophagus that allows the acid back from the stomach. A more serious cause of the acid could be a stomach ulcer. If you suffer continuously from poor digestion seek medical advice.

COMPRESSES

Prepare a bowl of hot water and place 4 drops of *BLEND* in it. Using a cotton cloth make a warm compress by soaking the cloth in the prepared water. Wring out and place across the top of the abdomen where the discomfort is experienced.

MASSAGE

Make up a bottle of Indigestion Treatment Oil by adding 12 drops of *BLEND* to 30ml of Sweet Almond Oil (see page 20).
Massage the Treatment Oil gently around the top of the abdomen. Do this between meals to help to calm the system down. Use gentle circular movements.

TISSUES

Put a 3 drops of *BLEND* onto a tissue. Inhale whenever the pain occurs. Take deep slow breathes.

LIFE STYLE

Spend 20 minutes winding down before eating and 20 minutes to allow digestion of the food after eating. This can make a great difference to the amount of discomfort you experience. Also eat slowly and deliberately chewing all your food thoroughly as this is the first part of the digestive action and one that you can control. Don't smoke - this irritates the stomach lining.
Try to reduce your stress level to a minimum.

DIET

Cut out fatty foods and those that contain food additives and spices. Eat small and regular meals.
Avoid aspirin as it harms the stomach lining.

☐ esters	21.2%
■ aliphatic aldehydes	1.0%
☐ ketones	2.5%
☐ sesquiterpenes	12.6%
■ lactones and coumarins	1.3%
☐ remainder	3.8%
☐ oxides	2.3%
☐ acids	trace
■ aromatic aldehydes	0.3%
☐ monoterpenes	19.5%
■ alcohols	34.7%
■ phenols, phe.ethers	0.8%

CCP of BLEND RECIPE

 🌢 *Lavender True* (lavandula angustifolia)

 🌢 *Tea Tree* (melaleuca alternifolia)

 🌢 *Bergamot* (citrus bergamia)

 🌢 *Myrrh* (commiphora myrrha)

Lavender True is excellent for the regeneration of skin cells. It heals wounds and scars and is on the whole a calming oil.

Tea Tree is strongly antiseptic which helps to protect the wound from infection.

Bergamot calms anxiety. It also assists skin to heal. It can be most helpful at combating depression.

Myrrh has a good drying effect on the skin. It will help the skin heal and also is calming to the nervous system.

All the chemical families are present in this blend with the esters, sesquiterpenes, monoterpenes and alcohols being the largest proportions.

Chemical constituents to be found in the blend may include:

■ linalyl acetate, lavandulyl acetate	■ α-pinene, β-pinene, γ–terpinene, α-terpinene, p-cymene
☐ cadinene, β-caryophyllene, elemene	■ α-terpineol, linalool, geraniol, myrrh alcohols, terpinen-4-ol, borneol, lavandulol

BLEND

10 drops *Lavender True*
10 drops *Tea Tree*
10 drops *Bergamot*
10 drops *Myrrh*
40 drops *BLEND*

Make up your *BLEND* using the quantities above - store in a small dark glass bottle fitted with a dropper (see page 20).

WATER SPRAY

Put 2 drops of the *BLEND* into a small cup of warm water. Put this into a fine water sprayer. If possible keep the wound open to the air and spray the ulcer regularly. When it is necessary to cover the ulcer for protection or for sleeping take a melamine dressing and before laying it over the ulcer spray it with the Treatment Water.
Make up a fresh cup of Treatment Water each day.
Persevere with this treatment keeping the ulcer open to the air when possible.
It may sting a little when you spray the ulcer.
Ulcers are very persistent, treatment will take 1-2 months to work.
Take great care of the wound area.

BATHS

If your doctor allows you to bath then add 8 drops of the *BLEND* to your bath water. This will keep the wound antiseptic.

COMPRESSES

Add 12 drops of the *BLEND* to 30ml of calendula oil. Gently massage a little of this Treatment Oil into the leg surrounding the wound. Allow a little of it to run onto the wound but do not actually touch the wound. Cut a soft cotton sheet to form a wadding to lay over the wound. Prepare some Treatment Water by putting 8 drops of *BLEND* into a basin of warm water. Soak the wadding in the treatment water. Squeeze out the wadding and lay it gently over the wound. Wrap cling film around the leg to hold the compress in place. Wrap a towel round to keep the warmth in. Leave in place for at least half an hour and longer if possible. The warmth encourages the circulation and helps the oils to penetrate the skin.

DRINK

Put one teaspoon of honey into a cup of hot water, add 1 drop of *Mint Peppermint* (mentha piperita).
Sip this drink slowly concentrating on relaxing. Rest with your feet raised.

FOOT MASSAGE

To help the circulation a daily foot massage is highly recommended. If possible book a treatment with a qualified reflexologist.

DIET

Take Zinc, Vitamins E, C, D, also beta-carotene(A) and garlic tablets. Cook with plenty of garlic and onions. Reduce intake of dairy products Drink herbal teas. Eat raw parsley.

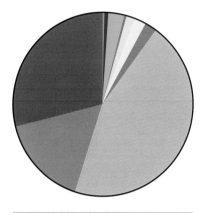

esters	0.2%
aliphatic aldehydes	0.5%
ketones	trace%
sesquiterpenes	3.3%
lactones and coumarins	0.2%
remainder	1.5%
oxides	2.3%
acids	trace
aromatic aldehydes	1.7%
monoterpenes	45.7%
alcohols	16.0%
phenols, phe.ethers	28.6%

CCP of BLEND RECIPE

  Cinnamon Leaf (cinnamomum zeylanicum)

  Grapefruit (citrus paradisi)

  Tea Tree (melaleuca alternifolia)

Cinnamon Leaf is antiviral, bactericidal, antioxidant, and a stimulant. It acts as a blood purifier. It is a powerful oil and is always used with care - avoid in pregnancy. The aroma is musty sweet and sharp.

Grapefruit has a sharp refreshing aroma. It is a very steadying oil and can be used to alleviate stress headaches and migraine attacks. It is excellent for local infections and congested skin.

Tea Tree is antiviral and strongly bactericidal. It is an immune system tonic and stimulates the body's healing processes. Extensively used in aboriginal medicine - excellent for treating infected wounds.

Chemical constituents to be found in the blend may include:

- benzyl benzoate, benzyl acetate, cinnamyl acetate, geranyl acetate
- citronellal, citral, sinensal
- β-caryophyllene, cadinene aromadendrene, viridiflorene
- auraptene, limettin
- 1.8-cineole, 1.4-cineole
- cinnamaldehyde, methyl vanillin
- α-pinene, α-terpinene, γ-terpinene p-cymene, limonene, terpinolene
- terpinen-4-ol, α-terpineol, globulol, geraniol, linalool, paradisiol, borneol
- eugenol, safrole, aceteugenol

BLEND

10 drops	*Cinnamon Leaf*
10 drops	*Grapefruit*
10 drops	*Tea Tree*
30 drops	*BLEND*

Make up your *BLEND* using the quantities above - store in a small dark glass bottle fitted with a dropper (see page 20).

AILMENT

Measles is a very common and contagious disease. The virus is transferred by airborne droplets and saliva. The incubation period is 7 to 14 days and the first symptoms to appear are a running nose and eyes followed by a sore throat and fever. Small red spots with white centres appear on the inside of the mouth - these are known as Kopliks spots. On the 4th day the blotchy skin rash spreads down the body starting from the face. The virus will run its course over the next 7 to 14 days. The dangerous aspect of measles is the fear of secondary infections. The body is particularly vulnerable to such complications as bronchitis, pneumonia, and ear infections that can lead to deafness.
It is necessary to take every precaution to prevent the sufferer becoming infected by other illnesses.

ROOM SPRAY

Add 5 drops of *BLEND* per litre of water and fill up a plant spray. Spray all the rooms in the house, including the sick room. This is a precaution to keep secondary infections at bay.

BODY LOTION

Make up a bottle of Measles Treatment Lotion by adding 5 drops of *Chamomile Roman* and 5 drops of *Lavender True* to 100ml of Calamine Lotion.
Shake the bottle well and apply gently all over the rash to ease the discomfort.

BATHS

Put 4 drops of *Chamomile Roman* in the bath.

TREATMENT

Keep the sufferer in bed for a few days and isolated from others as far as possible. It can help to keep the room slightly darkened as the eyes can be sensitive to light.
Measles is mainly a childhood disease and an attack builds up immunity. A vaccine was introduced in the 1960's which has reduced the reported cases of the disease considerably. Adult sufferers are likely to feel quite ill and need to take care from contracting any secondary infections.

DIET

Take Vitamin C 1000mgs per day. Stick to a light, easy to digest, diet. Drink 8 glasses of mineral water a day.

Menopause

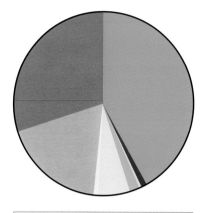

☐ esters	42.0%
■ aliphatic aldehydes	1.0%
☐ ketones	0.3%
☐ sesquiterpenes	2.0%
■ lactones and coumarins	trace
☐ remainder	5.8%
☐ oxides	0.4%
☐ acids	trace
■ aromatic aldehydes	
▨ monoterpenes	18.5%
▨ alcohols	30.0%
■ phenols, phe.ethers	trace

CCP of BLEND RECIPE

  Orange Blossom Neroli (citrus aurantium amara)

  Clary Sage (salvia sclarea)

Orange Blossom Neroli is analgesic, aphrodisiac and antiageing. The aroma is haunting and beautiful. The oil is very powerful for emotional problems. It has a balancing effect and is recommended for both menopausal problems and pre-menstrual tension.

Clary Sage is often called a woman's oil because of its oestrogen like action. It is calming, sedative and lowers blood pressure. The aroma is nutty and earthy. It is particularly recommended for menopausal problems.
Because of its hormone-like action avoid in cases of hormone related cancers. Also avoid in pregnancy and do not use if alcohol has been consumed.

Chemical constituents to be found in the blend may include:

☐ methyl anthranilate, linalyl acetate, geranyl acetate, neryl acetate
■ caryophyllenal
☐ jasmone, thujone, camphor
☐ caryophyllene, germacrene, bourbonene
☐ indole

☐ 1.8-cineole, caryophyllene oxide
☐ phenylacetic acid
☐ α-pinene, β-pinene, myrcene, limonene, phellandrene
▨ linalool, sclareol, α-terpineol, nerol, α-bisabolol, geraniol, nerolidol, benzyl alcohol, phenylethyl alcohol
■ methyl hexyl ether

BLEND

20 drops	*Orange Blossom Neroli*
20 drops	*Clary Sage*
40 drops	*BLEND*

Make up your *BLEND* using the quantities above - store in a small dark glass bottle fitted with a dropper (see page 20).

AILMENT

The menopause is not an ailment as such - it is just a natural ageing process. The ovaries cease to release an egg cell each month as the pituitary gland's and ovary's hormones change. The normal age for the menopause falls between 40 and 50 years old but there are many exceptions to this. Some women suffer extremely early onset of the menopause.

For many women the 'change of life' as it is called causes no problems whatsoever. For others the change proves quite distressing.

Actual physical phenomenon are the occurrence of 'hot flushes'. Not everybody experiences these and they normally cease after a few months and are mainly just an irritating discomfort. The more serious physical change in the body is the gradual loss of density from the bones that can lead to osteoporosis in later years. If there is a family history of bad osteoporosis it may be advisable to take Hormone Replacement Therapy (HRT) for a few years. Take medical advice on this. The emotional reaction to the hormonal change in the body is more complicated to deal with. Some women suffer depression which may be due not so much to the change of hormones as to the change of life style. Such things as all the children leaving home, new career patterns and so on all occur at this time.

MASSAGE

Make up a bottle of Menopause Treatment Oil by adding 12 drops of *BLEND* to 30ml of Sweet Almond Oil (see page 20).

Get a friend to give you a full body massage with this Treatment Oil at least once a week. Better still treat yourself to a regular visit to an aromatherapist. Taking time out for yourself will help tremendously with feelings of depression that can occur as you adjust to new life styles. The oils will work gently to restore a hormonal balance and the aromatherapist's experience and advice will help you understand why you are experiencing problems.

BATHS

Put 8 drops of *BLEND* in your bath. Soak and relax.

LIFE STYLE

Major desire at this time is to feel 'needed'. Work on positive ways of achieving this with new activities.

TISSUES

Put 1 drop of *Mint Peppermint* on a tissue. Inhale during 'hot flushes'.

DIET

Muti-vitamin tablets. Drink plenty of mineral water.

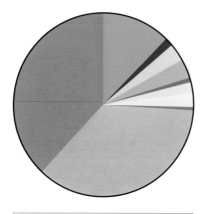

☐ esters	12.3%
■ aliphatic aldehydes	1.0%
☐ ketones	3.0%
☐ sesquiterpenes	3.3%
■ lactones and coumarins	0.6%
☐ remainder	2.2%
☐ oxides	2.3%
☐ acids	trace
■ aromatic aldehydes	0.3%
☐ monoterpenes	36.8%
■ alcohols	38.2%
■ phenols, phe.ethers	trace

CCP of BLEND RECIPE

 🌢 *Tea Tree* (melaleuca alternifolia)

  🌢 *Lavender True* (lavandula angustifolia)

 🌢 *Coriander* (coriandrum sativum)

 🌢 *Lemon* (citrus limon)

Tea Tree is antiviral, strongly bactericidal, decongestant and an immune system stimulant.

Lavender True is antiviral, analgesic, calming and balancing. It will help alleviate headaches and discomfort.

Coriander is analgesic and antiviral. It has a comforting sweet spicy woody aroma which blends well with the other oils.

Lemon is a decongestant and cleanses the body systems.

Chemical constituents to be found in the blend may include:

- ☐ linalyl acetate, geranyl acetate, neryl acetate, terpinyl acetate
- ■ citral, citronellal, nonanal, octanal,
- ☐ octanone, camphor, carvone
- ☐ β-bisabolene, α-bergamotene aromadendrene, viridiflorene
- ■ bergaptene, bergamottin coumarin, umbelliferone

- ☐ 1.8-cineole, linalool oxide
- ■ cuminaldehyde, benzaldehyde
- ☐ α-pinene, α-terpinene, γ-terpinene terpinolene, p-cymene, myrcene limonene, sabinene
- ■ terpinen-4-ol, α-terpineol, linalool, borneol, geraniol, lavandulol
- ■ anethole

BLEND

10 drops *Tea Tree*
10 drops *Lavender True*
10 drops *Coriander*
10 drops *Lemon*
40 drops *BLEND*

Make up your *BLEND* using the quantities above - store in a small dark glass bottle fitted with a dropper (see page 20).

AILMENT

Mumps is a common virus disease that most people get during childhood. The virus is similar to an influenza virus and is airborne. The first signs of mumps appear 2 to 4 weeks after exposure to the virus. It starts with a mild temperature and then the parotid salivary glands swell up painfully. This shows as an egg shaped swelling in front of the ear over the angle of the jaw bone. Sometimes the face just swells on the one side. The swelling usually subsides after a day or two. Occasionally the virus attacks other salivary glands and less often the testes or pancreas. As with most virus infections the nervous system may become involved. Earache often accompanies mumps and is particularly painful when eating. Normally the symptoms are mild and short lived.
If contracted as an adult it can cause sterility in men and there have been cases where diabetes was triggered. However these are rare occurrences.

ROOM SPRAY

Add 5 drops of *BLEND* per pint of water and fill up a plant spray. Spray rooms in the house and especially in the sick room.

APPLICATION

Make up a bottle of Mumps Treatment Oil by adding 12 drops of *BLEND* to 30ml of Sweet Almond Oil (see page 20).
Apply the treatment oil gently and carefully to the sore area. Also apply to the back of the neck and the abdominal area. Repeat the application 3 times daily.

TREATMENT

A few days rest are advisable to give the body support to deal with the virus. It will take its course. The oils will help with the pain and discomfort. Take mild pain killers if necessary.

DIET

The dryness in the mouth can be helped with a mouth wash.
Easy to eat foods are a good idea because of the pain in the jaw.
Soups and easy to digest foods.
Avoid any acid drinks such as orange juice.
Take supplements to boost the immune system.
Drink plenty of spring water.

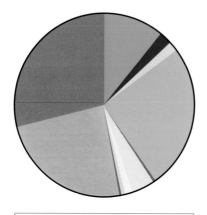

■ esters	10.8%
■ aliphatic aldehydes	2.2%
□ ketones	1.6%
■ sesquiterpenes	25.6%
■ lactones and coumarins	0.1%
□ remainder	4.9%
□ oxides	1.1%
□ acids	0.5%
■ aromatic aldehydes	0.2%
■ monoterpenes	23.8%
■ alcohols	29.2%
■ phenols, phe.ethers	trace

CCP of BLEND RECIPE

  Lavender True (lavandula angustifolia)

  Cypress (cupressus sempervirens)

  Sandalwood (santalum album)

  Ginger (zingiber officinale)

Lavender True is an antiinflammatory and an analgesic. It is a soothing and balancing oil.

Cypress balances the sympathetic nerve system. It is a decongestant and recommended for rheumatism.

Sandalwood is an antiinflammatory and helpful for lumbago.

Ginger is an analgesic, good for arthritis and back pains - a warming oil.

Chemical constituents to be found in the blend may include:

■ linalyl acetate, lavandulyl acetate
  α-terpinyl acetate, terpinen-4-yl acetate
■ citral, geranial, citronellal
□ octanone, camphor, santalone
  gingerone
■ β-caryophyllene, cedrene, santalenes,
  β-sesquiphellandrene, zingiberene
■ coumarin, umbelliferone

□ 1.8-cineole, manoyl oxide
  linalool oxide, caryophyllene oxide
□ nortricycloekasantalic acid
■ cuminaldehyde, benzaldehyde
■ camphene, limonene, α-pinene,
  β-pinene, Δ3-carene, p-cymene,
■ terpinen-4-ol, α-terpineol, linalool,
  borneol, geraniol, lavandulol
  sabinol, cedrol, santalols, gingerol

BLEND

8 drops	*Lavender True*
8 drops	*Cypress*
8 drops	*Sandalwood*
16 drops	*Ginger*
40 drops	*BLEND*

Make up your *BLEND* using the quantities above - store in a small dark glass bottle fitted with a dropper (see page 20).

AILMENT

Osteoarthritis is the degeneration of joints with some loss of the almost frictionless cartilage lining and the formation of rough deposits of bone. It is an inevitable ageing process but can occur in middle age if joints have been subjected to abnormal use or pressure. Such pressure can be caused by something as simple as poor posture, injury or athletic activities can trigger the condition. At first there are no symptoms of the cartilage loss but it first shows up as discomfort, pain and loss of movement.

If the pain becomes chronic and severe sometimes the only way to get relief from it is to undergo surgery. The Hip Replacement operation has brought relief to countless sufferers giving them back a quality of life free of pain and with mobility restored. Some operations 'fix' the painful joint. In this case the mobility is lost but the pain also vanishes.

BATHS

Put 8 drops of *BLEND* in your bath. Soak and relax. This will help the pain.

MASSAGE

Make up a bottle of Osteoarthritis Treatment Oil by adding 12 drops of *BLEND* to 30ml of Sweet Almond Oil (see page 20).
Massage the Treatment Oil gently around the affected joints. With osteoarthritis the connective tissue around the joint thickens and fluid may fill the joint. The essential oils will help to disperse this fluid. Repeat the massage 2 or 3 times daily.

TREATMENT

The degeneration of the joint cartilage can start quite innocently the only symptoms being an occasional ache an stiffness. However a more ominous 'creaking' sound when the joint is moved heralds the onset of more breakdown of movement. One thing that is essential is to make sure that you keep the joint moving every day otherwise immobility can set in.
If a joint is particularly painful make up a small 30ml pot of cream and add 12 drops of *Mint Peppermint* to it. Apply the ointment around the painful joint the *Mint Peppermint* will act as a local anaesthetic for a while.

DIET

Drink plenty of mineral water.
Cod liver oil capsules daily.
Fresh fruits and vegetables.
It is worth consulting a diet expert and having a personal food plan built up.

☐ esters	27.6%
■ aliphatic aldehydes	3.0%
☐ ketones	3.9%
☐ sesquiterpenes	7.3%
■ lactones and coumarins	0.6%
☐ remainder	2.0%
☐ oxides	2.8%
☐ acids	trace
■ aromatic aldehydes	
☐ monoterpenes	31.0%
☐ alcohols	21.8%
■ phenols, phe.ethers	trace

CCP of BLEND RECIPE

 ◊ *Yarrow* (achillea millefolium)

 ◊◊◊ *Chamomile Roman* (chamaemelum nobile)

 ◊◊◊ *Geranium* (pelargonium graveolens)

 ◊◊◊ *Lemon* (citrus limon)

Yarrow is antispasmodic and decongestant. A good women's oil. It should be avoided in pregnancy.

Chamomile Roman is antispasmodic, calming and soothing.

Geranium is analgesic, helps with anxiety and generally balances the body.

Lemon is antispasmodic, calming and clarifying. It lowers blood pressure and generally cleanses the body.

Chemical constituents to be found in the blend may include:

- ▦ bornyl acetate, angelates, tiglates, neryl acetate, citronellyl formate
- ■ citral, citronellal, nonanal
- ☐ isoartemisia, camphor, pinocarvone menthone, thujone
- ▦ chamazulene, caryophyllene, germacrene, dihydroazulene β-bisabolene, α-bergamotene
- ■ achilline, bergaptene, bergamottin
- ☐ 1.8-cineole, *cis*-rose oxide
- ▦ limonene, α-pinene, β-pinene, γ-terpinene, *p*-cymene, sabinene, myrcene, camphene
- ▦ citronellol, geraniol, linalool
- ■ eugenol

BLEND

4 drops *Yarrow*
12 drops *Chamomile Roman*
12 drops *Geranium*
12 drops *Lemon*
40 drops *BLEND*

Make up your *BLEND* using the quantities above - store in a small dark glass bottle fitted with a dropper (see page 20).

AILMENT

Heavy bleeding during the monthly menstruation, or clotting in the normal flow or irregular bleeding at any time of the month is known as menorrhagia.
If you are a chronic sufferer of any of these conditions you need to seek advice to track down the causes. Uterine bleeding can be a sign of uterine cancer or of a fibrous growth in the womb. It is a simple minor operation for the hospital to check your womb and give a clear diagnostic report.
The occasional occurrence of the conditions is often due to a stressful life style and slight hormonal imbalance.

TREATMENT

Make up a bottle of Heavy Periods Treatment Oil by adding 12 drops of *BLEND* to 30ml of Sweet Almond Oil (see page 20).
Take time out daily to massage your abdomen and lower back with the Treatment Oil.
Also organise to rest for 30 minutes in the middle of the day with your feet raised.

LIFE STYLE

Make a plan of a regular routine for the whole month. Time table the massage sessions and rest sessions. It is not so much the length of time for each session that is so important as the regularity of them. The body needs to establish a peaceful rhythm in order to function effectively.
Join a yoga or meditation class and learn the art of relaxation.
Treat yourself to a monthly appointment with a qualified aromatherapist or reflexologist. They will help you establish a plan.

BATHS

Put 8 drops of *BLEND* in your bath. Soak and relax.

VAPOURISER

Put 4 drops of *BLEND* in a vapouriser in any room that you are working in. The molecules of oil will circulate and have a calming effect.

DIET

Eat plenty of green leafy vegetables for their iron content.

Daily Supplements
Multi-vitamin/mineral tablet
Vitamin B6 100mgs
Vitamin C 1000mgs
Oil of Evening Primrose as per container.

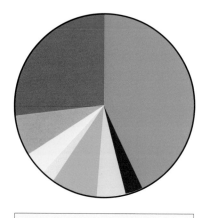

▨ esters	43.4%
■ aliphatic aldehydes	2.9%
☐ ketones	5.3%
▨ sesquiterpenes	8.6%
■ lactones and coumarins	trace
☐ remainder	2.0%
☐ oxides	4.1%
☐ acids	trace
■ aromatic aldehydes	
▨ monoterpenes	6.7%
■ alcohols	27.0%
■ phenols, phe.ethers	trace

CCP of BLEND RECIPE

 𐎖 *Yarrow* (achillea millefolium)

 𐎖𐎖𐎖𐎖 *Chamomile Roman* (chamaemelum nobile)

 𐎖𐎖𐎖 *Geranium* (pelargonium graveolens)

Yarrow is hormone like, stimulates secretions and is a good women's oil. Do not use during pregnancy. It is recommended for fibroids, ovaries, period problems and prolapse.

Chamomile Roman is a gentle calming oil. It will help anxiety and soothes the system. It is recommended for helping with the lack of periods (amenorrhoea) and nervous menstrual problems.

Geranium regulates hormone functions and generally balances the body. It helps with breast congestion, candida, painful periods, pmt and uterine haemorrhage.

Chemical constituents to be found in the blend may include:

▨ bornyl acetate, citronellyl formate, angelates, tiglates, butyrates
■ citral
☐ isoartemisia, camphor, thujone pinocarvone, menthone
☐ chamazulene, caryophyllene, germacrene, dihydroazulene

■ achilline
☐ 1.8-cineole, *cis*-rose oxide
▧ limonene, α-pinene, β-pinene, sabinene, camphene, myrcene
▨ citronellol, geraniol, linalool farnesol, nerolidol, α-terpineol
■ eugenol

BLEND

5 drops	*Yarrow*
20 drops	*Chamomile Roman*
15 drops	*Geranium*
40 drops	*BLEND*

Make up your *BLEND* using the quantities above - store in a small dark glass bottle fitted with a dropper (see page 20).

AILMENT

The condition of the menstrual cycle stopping is called amenorrhoea. The menstrual cycle may cease due to a range of causes. A common cause is an emotional upset or even a physical shock. More serious causes include disease of the ovaries, some disturbance of the pituitary gland and anorexia.

One of the problems with restoring the cycle is that anxiety about a lack of periods is in itself an emotional upset. As with so many of the hormonal balances within the body it is necessary to remove as much stress from daily life as possible in order to give the body a chance to establish its correct rhythm.

During pregnancy it is natural that the menstrual cycle ceases. This is medically called secondary amenorrhoea and should not be confused the condition being discussed here which to be precise is called primary amenorrhoea.

The menstrual cycle usually starts from the age of 13 years onwards although for some girls it is earlier. However for some girls it starts much later. A lack of periods will often right itself when the sufferer's quality of life improves and/or their general health improves.

TREATMENT

The best advice is to try keep your anxiety about the condition to a minimum. If you are feeling well in yourself the chances are that the body will restore its own rhythm. Essential oils are very helpful in balancing the endocrine system.

MASSAGE

Make up a bottle of Lack of Periods Treatment Oil by adding 12 drops of *BLEND* to 30ml of Sweet Almond Oil (see page 20).

Massage the abdomen and lower back with the Treatment Oil 3 or 4 times a week.

Book a monthly appointment with an aromatherapist who will be able to help you with the anxiety that you may be feeling.

BATHS

Put 8 drops of *BLEND* in your bath. Take your daily bath before going to bed. The oils will help to give you a peaceful sleep.

LIFE STYLE

Consult the list of life's most stressful situations in the Appendix and consider how you can reduce stress in your life. Yoga classes may help.

DIET

Daily Supplements
Multi-vitamin/mineral tablet
Vitamin B6 100mgs
Vitamin C 1000mgs

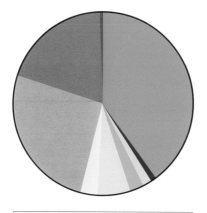

☐	esters	39.8%
■	aliphatic aldehydes	1.1%
☐	ketones	1.5%
▨	sesquiterpenes	2.5%
■	lactones and coumarins	trace
☐	remainder	5.7%
☐	oxides	2.8%
☐	acids	trace
▨	aromatic aldehydes	
▨	monoterpenes	26.3%
▨	alcohols	20.0%
■	phenols, phe.ethers	0.3%

CCP of BLEND RECIPE

  Rose Otto (rosa damascena)

  Cypress (cupressus sempervirens)

 Chamomile Roman (chamaemelum nobile)

Rose Otto is hormone like it regulates and stimulates the pituitary gland. It is antispasmodic, balancing and calming. The aroma is sweet, heavenly and flowery. It is a woman's oil that calms, relieves tension and feelings of inadequacy.

Cypress regulates the ovarian function and balances the sympathetic nerve system. It is recommended for irregular periods, menopause and pmt. The aroma is clear, woody and spicy.

Chamomile Roman is highly respected for its calming influence on all systems. It balances the menstrual cycle and helps with anaemia. The aroma is earthy, fruity and apple like.

Chemical constituents to be found in the blend may include:

- ▨ angelates, α-terpinyl acetate, tiglates, citronellyl acetate, geranyl acetate,
- ■ neral
- ☐ pinocarvone
- ▨ chamazulene, caryophyllene cedrene, cadinene
- I☐ damascenone

- ☐ 1.8-cineole, manoyl oxide,rose oxide
- ▨ α-pinene, β-pinene, Δ3-carene , p-cymene, camphene, limonene stearoptene, camphene, ocimene
- ▨ citronellol, geraniol, nerol, sabinol, α-terpineol, *trans*-pinocarveol
- ■ methyl eugenol

BLEND

10 drops *Rose Otto*
10 drops *Cypress*
20 drops *Chamomile Roman*
40 drops *BLEND*

Make up your *BLEND* using the quantities above - store in a small dark glass bottle fitted with a dropper (see page 20).

AILMENT

Many women are affected by menstrual pain just before and during their period.
The uterine cramps and sets up lower back and abdomen pains sometimes so severe that it is necessary to lie down until they ease up.
The whole episode can be made much worse if the situation is very stressful and there is no opportunity for relaxing and dealing with it.
If the severe pains are experienced every month for several days it is wise to seek medical advice just in case it is a symptom of a more serious problem.

TREATMENT

The best way to try and tackle this problem is to take some preventative measures.
The daily massage treatment described below should commence 14 days before your period is due.
Keep your diary as clear as possible over the dates of your period. This will lift the level of anxiety that you may feel as the dates approach. Fear of pain can actually trigger a pain reaction.

MASSAGE

Make up a bottle of Painful Periods Treatment Oil by adding 12 drops of *BLEND* to 30ml of Sweet Almond Oil (see page 20).
Apply the Treatment Oil each night to the small of the back and the lower abdomen. Gently massage over the abdomen with circular clockwise strokes.

BATHS

Put 8 drops of *BLEND* in your bath. Soak and relax.

LIFE STYLE

Make a plan to spend your next 'period week' in a very relaxed fashion.
For instance - get a really interesting book from the library and plan some peaceful evenings curled up on a comfortable sofa with your book and some relaxing music.
Or dig out your favourite video and buy in your favourite menu and plan an evening of relaxed viewing.
Whatever you choose the whole idea is to spoil yourself and let the rest of the world take care of itself for a few days.

DIET

Drink plenty of spring water.
Keep to a light and easily digestible foods during the period days.
Evening Primrose Tablets as per container.

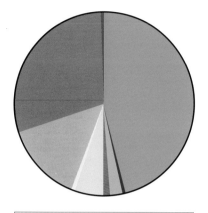

▨ esters	46.0%
■ aliphatic aldehydes	0.4%
☐ ketones	trace
▨ sesquiterpenes	2.4%
■ lactones and coumarins	1.3%
☐ remainder	5.4%
☐ oxides	0.5%
☐ acids	trace
■ aromatic aldehydes	
▨ monoterpenes	14.2%
▨ alcohols	29.4%
■ phenols, phe.ethers	0.4%

CCP of BLEND RECIPE

  Clary Sage (salvia sclarea)

  Rose Otto (rosa damascena)

  Bergamot (citrus bergamia)

Clary Sage is calming and a sedative. It helps with panic attacks and depression. It is oestrogen like and should be avoided in cases of hormone related cancers. Recommended for menopausal problems.

Rose Otto is balancing, calming and cheering. It increases confidence and is recommended for pmt. It regulates the endocrine system and is hormone like in its action. Believed to release dopamine.

Bergamot is antispasmodic and calming. Especially recommended for calming agitation and anxiety. This oil is often the first choice in cases of depression. The aroma is a light, refreshing citrus note. It is used in Earl Grey tea.

Chemical constituents to be found in the blend may include:

- ▨ linalyl acetate, geranyl acetate, neryl acetate, citronellyl acetate
- ■ caryophyllenal, citral
- ☐ thujone, camphor
- ▨ caryophyllene, germacrene, bourbonene, β-bisabolene
- ■ bergaptene

- ☐ damascenone
- ☐ 1.8-cineole, rose oxide
- ▨ β-pinene, γ-terpinene, α-terpinene, limonene, stearoptene, camphene
- ▨ linalool, sclareol, α-terpineol, citronellol, geraniol, farnesol, nerol
- ■ methyl hexyl ether, methyl eugenol

BLEND

20 drops *Clary Sage*
10 drops *Rose Otto*
10 drops *Bergamot*
40 drops *BLEND*

Make up your *BLEND* using the quantities above - store in a small dark glass bottle fitted with a dropper (see page 20).

AILMENT

Premenstrual tension - pmt is caused by the change in the balance of female hormones during the menstrual cycle. Troublesome but mainly harmless symptoms become evident in the run up to a period. Unfortunately this can mean that some women are coping with them for 50% of the month. Problems include fluid retention, swollen joints, food and alcohol cravings, weight gain, skin problems, weakness and headaches. Psychological reactions can manifest themselves in irritability, irrationality, decreased sex drive, insomnia, tearfulness and depression.

The reason for many of the symptoms is the drop in level of progesterone - this in turn causes the sugar and salt levels to rise which will lead to fluid retention. The hormonal balance in the body is a feed back system and it generally restores itself. As fluid retention will affect all the cells in the body including those in the brain this could be the main cause of the problems that arise both physically and mentally. Some women become so disturbed that they literally become another person for a day or two.

TREATMENT

With a regular cyclic disturbance such as this planning is all important. Try to organise your diary both at work and at home so that during the difficult days you do not attempt unreasonable tasks.
Discuss your problem openly with family and colleagues.

MASSAGE

Make up a bottle of Periods-pmt Treatment Oil by adding 12 drops of *BLEND* to 30ml of Almond Oil (see page 20).
Massage with the Treatment Oil is one of the most effective ways of helping your system balance itself. Massage all around your shoulders where the tension is likely to build up. Also massage your abdomen with circular clockwise strokes and finally massage the small of your back. Do this routine every night starting a fortnight before your period is due. Book a regular appointment with an aromatherapist who will also be able to personally advise you.

TISSUES / VAPOURISER

Put drops of *BLEND* on tissues and in your vaporiser as needed.

BATHS

Put 8 drops of *BLEND* in your baths.

DIET

Vitamin B6
Evening Primrose Oil

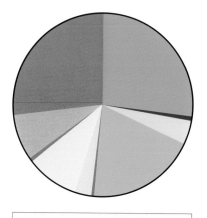

▨ esters	27.4%
▪ aliphatic aldehydes	0.6%
▫ ketones	4.2%
▨ sesquiterpenes	19.0%
▪ lactones and coumarins	0.2%
▫ remainder	3.2%
▫ oxides	9.6%
▫ acids	trace
▪ aromatic aldehydes	0.6%
▨ monoterpenes	8.2%
▨ alcohols	27.0%
▪ phenols, phe.ethers	trace

CCP of BLEND RECIPE

  Lavender True (lavandula angustifolia)

  Yarrow (achillea millefolium)

 Chamomile German (matricaria recutica)

Lavender True is excellent for the regeneration of skin cells. It heals wounds and scars and is on the whole a calming oil. Lower back massage helps dispel afterbirth. It is antiviral, antiseptic and a nervous system regulator.

Yarrow acts on the bone marrow and stimulates blood renewal. It is useful for varicose veins, lowers blood pressure and is a good decongestant. The aroma is sweet, spicy and camphorous.

Chamomile German is hormone like, temperature reducing and stimulates secretions. It is bactericidal and antiinflammatory - especially helpful for wounds, rashes and skin problems.

Chemical constituents to be found in the blend may include:

- ▨ linalyl acetate, geranyl acetate, lavandulyl acetate, bornyl acetate
- ▪ citral
- ▫ isoartemisia, camphor
- ▫ chamazulene, caryophyllene, germacrene, dihydroazulene
- ▪ coumarin, umbelliferone, achilline
- ▫ en-yn-dicycloether, *cis*-spiro-ether

- ▫ α-bisabolol oxide, 1.8-cineole
- ▨ cuminaldehyde, benzaldehyde
- ▨ α-pinene, β-pinene, sabinene, camphene, ocimene, limonene
- ▨ terpinen-4-ol, α-terpineol, linalool, borneol, geraniol, lavandulol α-bisabolol, cadinol
- ▪ eugenol

BLEND

24 drops	*Lavender True*
8 drops	*Yarrow*
8 drops	*Chamomile German*
40 drops	*BLEND*

Make up your *BLEND* using the quantities above - store in a small dark glass bottle fitted with a dropper (see page 20).

AILMENT

After the birth both mother and baby are adjusting to their new life style. Minor infections are fairly common and nature provides protection to a great extent during the early days. The baby inherits its mother's immunity for a while. In less developed countries mothers use the colostrum that flows from the breasts for 2 to 3 days after birth to heal minor infections. As the colostrum is rich in antibodies just dabbing a little on an infected area can clear infections such as cuts, sores and eye infections.

BATHS AND BIDETS

After birth the first priority is to keep the genital area scrupulously clean.This will prevent infections from starting up.
If you have a bidet you can use that to fully immerse the genital area. Otherwise use the bath and just fill to an appropriate level. Add 2 drops of *BLEND* to the bidet and 4 to 8 drops of *BLEND* to the bath depending on the level of water. Also add salt to the water as salt is a natural disinfectant. Use the bidet or bath at least 3 times a day. If you are suffering an infection in the wounds then make sure that you keep the area immersed for at least 5 minutes. This will give the oils time to be absorbed. Don't cheat on this - make the bathroom comfortably warm and rest in the water reading a book.

TREATMENT

Make up a bottle of Post-natal Treatment Oil by adding 6 drops of *BLEND* to 30ml of Sweet Almond Oil (see page 20).
Make up a pot of Post-natal Treatment Lotion by adding 6 drops of *BLEND* to 30ml of Lotion (see Carriers).
The Treatment Oil and the Treatment Lotion can be used throughout the baby's early months.
If the baby develops any skin rashes or small wounds of any kind just gently apply a little of the oil or lotion. You can also apply the Treatment Oil or Lotion to yourself. If you are experiencing a burning pain on passing urine due to postnatal soreness wash the area and just rub a little Treatment Oil around it. If the pain is really sharp a good trick is to rub a little vaseline on before you urinate. This protects the sore area from the acid in the urine.
Essential oils are excellent for helping skin and wounds to heal.

DIET

Eat light healthy diet with plenty of fresh vegetables and fruit. Perhaps not too much citrus fruit.
Be careful to keep your calcium level adequate.

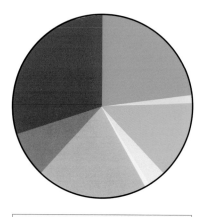

☐ esters	23.3%
■ aliphatic aldehydes	trace
☐ ketones	1.3%
☐ sesquiterpenes	13.3%
■ lactones and coumarins	trace
☐ remainder	2.8%
☐ oxides	0.8%
☐ acids	trace
■ aromatic aldehydes	trace
☐ monoterpenes	20.7%
☐ alcohols	7.7%
■ phenols, phe.ethers	30.1%

CCP of BLEND RECIPE

   Black Pepper (piper nigrum)

   Clove Bud (syzygium aromaticum)

   Clary Sage (salvia sclarea)

Black Pepper is analgesic and antispasmodic. It is recommended for aches and pains, rheumatism, rheumatoid arthritis and temporary paralysis. The aroma is sharp and spicy.

Clove Bud is analgesic, antispasmodic, an antioxidant and stimulating. It has hormone like properties and balances thyroid problems. The aroma is strong and spicy.

Clary Sage is antispasmodic, calming, a sedative and a tonic. It is oestrogen like and should be avoided in cases of hormone related cancers. Do not use if alcohol has been consumed.

Chemical constituents to be found in the blend may include:

☐ linalyl acetate, geranyl acetate, neryl acetate
■ caryophyllenal
☐ piperitone, dihydrocarvone camphor thujone
☐ β-caryophyllene, bisabolene germacrene, bourbonene, humulenes

☐ 1.8-cineole, caryophyllene oxide
☐ limonene, α-pinene, β-pinene, sabinene, terpinenes, myrcene, phellandrene, camphene, thujene
■ terpinen-4-ol, α-terpineol, linalool sclareol, α-bisabolol
■ myristicin, safrole, aceteugenol eugenol, methyl hexyl ether

BLEND

14 drops *Black Pepper*
14 drops *Clove Bud*
14 drops *Clary Sage*
42 drops *BLEND*

Make up your *BLEND* using the quantities above - store in a small dark glass bottle fitted with a dropper (see page 20).

AILMENT

Unlike osteoarthritis which is progressive and irreversible rheumatoid arthritis may come and go spontaneously. There is no sure cure and the underlying causes are not fully understood. Physical and emotional stresses may play some part in triggering an attack. The characteristic feature of an attack is a small knot of inflamed fibrous tissue often just under the skin. Any organ can be affected but the most common are the knuckle joints and the wrist. The inflammation may subside without inflicting much damage but if a chronic attack sets in then the joint may become damaged and eventually deformed. The inflammation causes the muscles around the joint to tighten and the cartilage may become damaged over time.

It is thought that for some reason the immune system sees some normal body cells as 'foreign bodies' and attacks them. Such a disease is classified as an autoimmune disease. Rheumatoid arthritis is more common in women than in men. The pain and inflammation can be helped with the essential oils. Very severe attacks may eventually need surgery to ease the deformities.

As the first attack of the condition often follows a virus infection or an illness it could well be linked to the functioning of the glands and hormones.

BATHS

Put 2 handfuls of Epsom Salts and 8 drops of *BLEND* in your bath. Bath daily giving yourself time to relax and soak in the comfort of the warm water.

MASSAGE

Make up a bottle of Rheumatoid Arthritis Treatment Oil by adding 12 drops of *BLEND* to 30ml of Sweet Almond Oil (see page 20). Massage the oil over your shoulders. Get a friend to give you a full body massage or even just a back massage at regular intervals. The oils will be absorbed into your blood stream and will help with the inflammation and pain. Gently apply a little Treatment Oil to affected joints.

DIET

If you are suffering from severe attacks it is worth taking some effort to check whether it is a food allergy that is triggering the attacks. If so you may be able to control the condition by following the correct diet.

It is probably best to seek professional help in setting up a closely monitored food plan.

You can try yourself by cutting your diet back to only a few items and then gradually including other items one at a time. You may be able to identify the culprit. Red meat sometimes seems to be the problem.

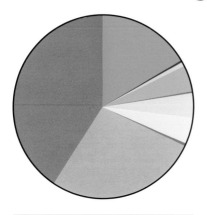

☐ esters	17.0%
■ aliphatic aldehydes	0.2%
☐ ketones	0.8%
☐ sesquiterpenes	4.6%
■ lactones and coumarins	0.1%
☐ remainder	3.9%
☐ oxides	4.6%
☐ acids	trace
■ aromatic aldehydes	0.2%
☐ monoterpenes	27.4%
■ alcohols	41.2%
■ phenols, phe.ethers	trace

CCP of BLEND RECIPE

   Lavender True (lavandula angustifolia)

   Tea Tree (melaleuca alternifolia)

   Thyme Common Sweet (thymus vulgaris linaloliferum)

Lavender True is excellent for the regeneration of skin cells. It heals wounds and scars and is on the whole a calming oil. It is recommended for arthritis, burns, radiography burns, eczema, herpes, psoriasis, spots and wounds.

Tea Tree is antifungal and strongly antiseptic and is recommended for athlete's foot, bites, boils, burns, radiography burns, cold sores, itching, mouth ulcers, ringworm, spots, sweaty feet, wounds.

Thyme Common Sweet is antioxidant, antifungal, antiinflammatory, antiseptic. It is recommended for acne, dry and wet eczema, muscular rheumatism, psoriasis and verrucas.

Chemical constituents to be found in the blend may include:

■ linalyl acetate, geranyl acetate, lavandulyl acetate
■ citral
☐ octanone, camphor
■ aromadendrene, viridiflorene, cadinene, β-caryophyllene
■ coumarin, umbelliferone

☐ 1.8-cineole, linalool oxide
■ cuminaldehyde, benzaldehyde
■ α-pinene, α-terpinene, γ-terpinene p-cymene, limonene, terpinolene, myrcene, ocimene, camphene
■ terpinen-4-ol, α-terpineol, linalool, borneol, lavandulol, globulol, viridiflorol

BLEND

8 drops	*Lavender True*
24 drops	*Tea Tree*
8 drops	*Thyme Common Sweet*
40 drops	*BLEND*

Make up your *BLEND* using the quantities above - store in a small dark glass bottle fitted with a dropper (see page 20).

AILMENT

Ringworm is one of the commonest skin diseases. The outer layer of the skin is infected with a microscopic fungus. Athlete's foot is one example of a strain of this fungus. With some types the fungus spreads out as a disc across the skin. The skin in the centre of the disc heals and the fungus moves outwards on the perimeter. This 'ring' appearance gives the condition its name. It can appear on the scalp, in the groin or as mentioned above on the feet. It can also appear elsewhere on the body. If small blisters occur this is an allergic reaction to the fungus. The nails of the fingers and the toes may harbour the fungus which causes them to become slightly deformed. If the fungus is in the scalp small areas of hair loss will be experienced. The fungus can be passed on from people and animals.

LIFE STYLE

Keep all towels and flannels isolated to prevent the infection spreading. If clothes have been in contact with the fungus add 4 drops of *BLEND* to the rinse water when you wash them. In a washing machine add 4 drops of *BLEND* to the softener that you use for the rinse cycle.

In the case of Athlete's foot avoid changing rooms and swimming pools until the condition has cleared.

APPLICATION

Apply 1 drop of *BLEND* to the affected area 3 times a day until it is clear. This should take about 10 days. Make up a bottle of Ringworm Treatment Oil by adding 12 drops of *BLEND* to 30ml of Sweet Almond Oil (see page 20).

After the fungus has cleared rub the Treatment Oil over the area where the infection was and this will stop it from starting up again. Do this daily for a week.

Watch out for any sign of the fungus returning and repeat the treatment immediately before it has a chance to become established.

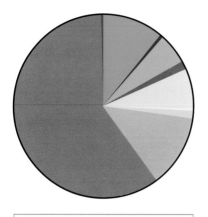

▦ esters	11.0%
■ aliphatic aldehydes	0.4%
☐ ketones	trace
▦ sesquiterpenes	5.4%
■ lactones and coumarins	1.3%
☐ remainder	7.6%
☐ oxides	0.1%
☐ acids	1.3%
■ aromatic aldehydes	
▦ monoterpenes	13.2%
■ alcohols	59.4%
■ phenols, phe.ethers	0.3%

CCP of BLEND RECIPE

  Sandalwood (santalum album)

  Rose Otto (rosa damascena)

 ◊ *Bergamot* (citrus bergamia)

Sandalwood is an aphrodisiac, calming and a tonic. It is recommended for impotence. Well known for bringing peaceful feelings - it is used for incenses and meditation..

Rose Otto is an aphrodisiac, antispasmodic, balancing and calming. It calms jealous feelings and increases confidence. It is recommended for frigidity and impotence.

Bergamot is widely used to calm agitation and panic attacks. It has a gentle action covering a wide range of therapeutic uses. The aroma is light and citrus which balances the rose and sandalwood aromas well.

Chemical constituents to be found in the blend may include:

▦ citronellyl acetate, geranyl acetate, neryl acetate, linalyl acetate
■ citral
☐ santalone
▦ santalenes, curcumenes, farnesene caryophyllene, β-bisabolene
▩ bergaptene
☐ damascenone

☐ rose oxide
☐ nortricycloekasantalic acid
▦ β-pinene, γ-terpinene, α-terpinene, limonene, stearoptene, camphene,
■ santalols, tricycloekasantalol, nerol, borneol, citronellol, geraniol, linalool, farnesol
■ methyl eugenol

BLEND

20 drops *Sandalwood*
10 drops *Rose Otto*
10 drops *Bergamot*
40 drops *BLEND*

Make up your *BLEND* using the quantities above - store in a small dark glass bottle fitted with a dropper (see page 20).

AILMENT

Inadequacy, real or imaginary is the commonest reason why people find their sex drive diminished. Frigidity is a lack of sexual desire that is normally applied to women but can equally apply to men. It is important to identify any physical conditions that prevent coitus. A man may be impotent either because he physically cannot achieve an erection due to some physical illness or because of emotional problems.

Sexual activity is usually depressed by general ill health anyway.

Most impotency and frigidity problems are caused by emotional states of mind. Lack of sex drive, rather than being due to any deep seated physchological childhood trauma, is often due simply to a shyness that either sex can suffer from, together with an inferiority complex about their sexual attractiveness. It is seldom that they find their partner sexually unattractive but more likely that they are discontent with their own physical appearance. Unfortunately their partner can easily misunderstand the problem and feel unnecessarily rejected. In such a case a vicious circle of misunderstanding can set up between the partners.

A woman is seldom roused as quickly as a man and as in nature an initial reluctance is part of the wooing process. Few couple achieve sexual harmony at once, although this is rarely admitted. Patience and understanding are essential ingredients in building a satisfying sexual relationship.

TREATMENT

Talk through any problem with your partner. Recognise each others needs and work together to resolve any hang ups. A warm and cosy atmosphere and plenty of time to build up to a climax will provide satisfaction to both partners.

MASSAGE

Make up a bottle of Sex Drive Problems Treatment Oil by adding 12 drops of *BLEND* to 30ml of Sweet Almond Oil (see page 20).

Quite separate from sexual encounters exchange body massages with your partner regularly. Such a massage should not be seeking any sexual response. It is essential that the partner receiving the massage can completely relax rather than be expected to make any response. The aim of the massage is to relax the mind and to create emotional confidence. The essential oils will lower feelings of anxiety and enhance feelings of self esteem.

VAPOURISER

Put 8 drops of *BLEND* in the vapouriser to create a relaxed environment.

■ esters	1.0%
■ aliphatic aldehydes	2.5%
□ ketones	1.0%
■ sesquiterpenes	29.3%
■ lactones and coumarins	
□ remainder	5.6%
□ oxides	1.4%
□ acids	trace
■ aromatic aldehydes	
■ monoterpenes	28.8%
■ alcohols	6.4%
■ phenols, phe.ethers	24.0%

CCP of BLEND RECIPE

 ♦♦♦♦   *Ginger* (zingiber officinale)

 ♦♦   *Nutmeg* (myristica fragrans)

 ♦♦   *Clove Bud* (syzygium aromaticum)

Ginger is analgesic and it helps to disperse blood clots. It is a warming oil that stimulates the blood circulation. The aroma is warm, pleasant and spicy. Used in many ancient remedies.

Nutmeg is invigorating to heart and circulation. Treat with care the myristicin can cause hallucinations. Avoid in pregnancy.

Clove Bud is analgesic, antispasmodic and stimulating. It raises blood pressure. Check for skin irritation. Used in traditional medicine for alleviating toothache. Used in many modern pharmaceuticals. The aroma is strong and spicy.

Chemical constituents to be found in the blend may include:

■ geranial, citronellal
□ gingerone
■ β-sesquiphellandrene, zingiberene, *ar*-curcumene, β-caryophyllene humulenes
□ 1.8-cineole, caryophyllene oxide, humulene oxide

▩ α-pinene, β-pinene, α-terpinene, γ-terpinene, sabinene, myrcene, limonene, camphene, *p*-cymene
■ citronellol, linalool, terpinen-4-ol, borneol, gingerol, geraniol
■ eugenol, isoeugenol, aceteugenol myristicin, elemicin, safrole

BLEND

20 drops *Ginger*
10 drops *Nutmeg*
10 drops *Clove Bud*
40 drops *BLEND*

Make up your *BLEND* using the quantities above - store in a small dark glass bottle fitted with a dropper (see page 20).

AILMENT

A sprain occurs when the fibres of the connective tissue are torn and damaged without a bone being broken or dislocated. Sometimes bleeding occurs. The damaged tissue causes swelling and is extremely painful. The body restricts the movement of the area because of the pain and this generally ensures that the movement is reduced such that the healing can take place. This is in contrast to the case of a broken bone which requires setting and plastering. If the pain and swelling from a suspected sprain does not disperse after a day or two there could well be a small fracture in the bone and it is wise to have the injury examined and scanned.

It is possible to sprain or strain any area of the body.

The treatment of a sprain with compresses will speed the recovery in most cases.

Rest the injury as far as possible.

COMPRESSES

For most sprains the following treatment is recommended. Prepare an ice cold bowl of water and add 5 drops of the *BLEND*. Make a compress out of clean cotton cloth. Soak the cloth in the prepared water, wring out and place around the injured area. Repeat this several times to start the cooling process and to allow the oils to penetrate the wound. Next use an icebag or even a 'frozen bag of peas' and place it on the injured area for twenty minutes. Once the swelling subsides and certainly by the next day you can start applying hot and cold compresses alternately. This will encourage the blood to circulate to the injured area and speed up the healing processes.

APPLICATION

Make up a bottle of Sprain Treatment Oil by adding 12 drops of *BLEND* to 30ml of Almond Oil (see Carriers). Just after the injury has occurred gently stroke the Treatment Oil around the area. As the sprain heals you can gradually increase pressure of the strokes. Again you want to encourage blood flow to the injury which together with the oils will speed the healing.

Sprains can take some time to completely heal, a period of 6 to 8 weeks is to be expected.

BATHS

Put 8 drops of *BLEND*. in your bath. Soak and relax in a warm bath to ease the pain.

▨ esters	34.0%
■ aliphatic aldehydes	1.0%
☐ ketones	3.0%
▨ sesquiterpenes	3.8%
■ lactones and coumarins	0.2%
▨ remainder	2.0%
☐ oxides	1.5%
☐ acids	
▨ aromatic aldehydes	0.8%
▨ monoterpenes	25.5%
▨ alcohols	28.2%
■ phenols, phe.ethers	trace

CCP of BLEND RECIPE

  Lavender True (lavandula angustifolia)

  Mandarin (citrus reticulata)

Lavender True is antifungal, antiinflammatory, antiseptic, a good cell regenerator. It is recommended for all kinds of skin damage such as stretch marks, burns, radiography burns, eczema, herpes, psoriasis,spots, wounds. The aroma is the comfortingly familiar lavender scent with its memories of warm summer days.

Mandarin is antiseptic, a cell regenerator.and excellent for preventing stretch marks. It acts on the endocrine system and is particularly useful in balancing the metabolic rate. The oil is calming and helps to break down fats, decrease flatulence and improve bile production. This fruit was given to the Mandarins as a mark of respect - hence its name. The aroma is sweet sharp and floral.

Chemical constituents to be found in the blend may include:

- ▨ linalyl acetate, geranyl acetate, lavandulyl acetate methyl anthranilate
- ■ decanal, sinensal, citral, citronellal
- ☐ octanone, camphor
- ▨ β-caryophyllene
- ■ coumarin, umbelliferone
- ☐ 1.8-cineole, linalool oxide

- ▨ cuminaldehyde, benzaldehyde
- ▨ γ-terpinene, limonene, pinenes, myrcene, *p*-cymene, ocimene
- ▨ linalool, geraniol, terpinen-4-ol α-terpineol, lavandulol citronellol, octanol, borneol
- ■ eugenol, thymol

BLEND

30 drops *Lavender True*
10 drops *Mandarin*
40 drops *BLEND*

Make up your *BLEND* using the quantities above - store in a small dark glass bottle fitted with a dropper (see page 20).

AILMENT

If the skin is stretched over long periods it looses some of its elasticity. This results in white silvery stretch marks appearing across the surface of the skin.
In pregnancy the areas at risk of stretch marks are the lower abdomen and the breasts. In adolescence many girls put on extra weight and stretch marks might show up on the thighs and breasts. Obesity of course will also cause this problem to occur. Essential oils cannot cure the damage once it has occurred but they can help the skin's appearance. By far the best approach is to take preventative measures against the forming of stretch marks.
The preventative treatment below will ensure that you do not develop stretch marks during pregnancy.

MASSAGE

Make up a bottle of Stretch Marks Treatment Oil by adding 12 drops of *BLEND* to 15ml of Sweet Almond Oil and 15ml of Calendula Oil (see Carriers).
To keep the skin in excellent condition during pregnancy apply the Treatment Oil to the lower abdomen and around the breasts every evening and morning. Start early in the pregnancy and certainly no later than the fourth month.

TREATMENT

For skin that is already damaged apply the Treatment Oil every day to improve the condition of the skin. If the stretch marks are due to being overweight do make every effort to tackle the problem. Consider joining a local slimming group such as Weight Watchers. Such a support group can help you with sensible food plans and the help of others who will understand how you are feeling.

ESSENTIAL OILS

Other essential oils that you can use for stretch marks are:

Frankincense (boswellia carteri)
Myrrh (commiphora molmol)
Geranium (perlargonium graveolens).

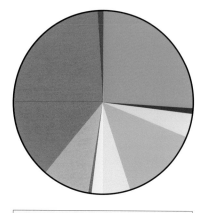

☐ esters	25.7%
■ aliphatic aldehydes	1.1%
☐ ketones	4.0%
▨ sesquiterpenes	14.9%
■ lactones and coumarins	0.2%
☐ remainder	4.0%
☐ oxides	2.1%
☐ acids	trace
■ aromatic aldehydes	0.6%
▨ monoterpenes	8.1%
▨ alcohols	38.4%
■ phenols, phe.ethers	0.9%

CCP of BLEND RECIPE

 𝛟𝛟𝛟𝛟 *Lavender True* (lavandula angustifolia)

  𝛟 *Tea Tree* (melaleuca alternifolia)

  𝛟𝛟 *Myrrh* (commiphora myrrha)

Lavender True is antifungal, antiinflammatory, antiseptic and an excellent cell regenerator. It is recommended for arthritis, burns, radiography burns, eczema, herpes, psoriasis, spots and wounds. It is generally a calming oil with excellent bactericidal and antiinflammatory properties.

Tea Tree is antifungal, antiinflammatory, strongly antiseptic and a parasiticide. It is recommended for athlete's foot, bites, boils, burns, radiography burns, cold sores, itching, mouth ulcers, ringworm, spots, sweaty feet and wounds.

Myrrh is bactericidal and antifungal. It has a good drying effect on the skin. It will help the skin heal and also is calming to the nervous system.

Chemical constituents to be found in the blend may include:

- ▨ linalyl acetate, geranyl acetate, lavandulyl acetate, myrrholic ester,
- ■ citral, 2-butanal
- ☐ octanone, camphor, curzerenone methyl isobutyl ketone
- ☐ aromadendrene, viridiflorene, cadinene, caryophyllene, elemene, heerabolene, cadinene, copaene
- ▨ coumarin, umbelliferone

- ☐ 1.8-cineole, linalool oxide
- ☐ myrrholic acid
- ▨ cinnamaldehyde, cuminaldehyde
- ▨ α-pinene, α-terpinene, γ-terpinene p-cymene, limonene, terpinolene, myrcene, ocimene, camphene
- ▨ terpinen-4-ol, α-terpineol, linalool, borneol, myrrh alcohols lavandulol
- ■ eugenol

BLEND

24 drops *Lavender True*
 6 drops *Tea Tree*
12 drops *Myrrh*
42 drops *BLEND*

Make up your *BLEND* using the quantities above - store in a small dark glass bottle fitted with a dropper (see page 20).

AILMENT

Thrush is an infection that commonly occurs in the mouth, intestines and vagina. It is triggered when the normal level of candida in the body is exceeded. Candida is a fungus related to the yeasts and is a normal part of the body's mucous membranes. If the general bacterial balance of the body is maintained then the growth of candida is suppressed to the correct level. If the bacterial level is reduced, say by a course of antibiotics, then the level of candida will increase and an attack of thrush may result.

In the mouth thrush can be recognised as white patches. In the vagina it can become quite troublesome and uncomfortable. The area will become itchy and sore and a thick white discharge may set up. The infection can be passed by a sexual partner and once it occurs both partners need to take steps to prevent further outbreaks or it can pass back and forth between them. Over weight people may also be prone to the condition as it settles in warm moist folds of the body. Babies also show the infection in their mouths and in an attack of nappy rash.

MOUTH WASH

For oral thrush put 1 drop of *BLEND* in a glass of warm boiled water, swish round well. Use as a mouth wash 3 times a day.

APPLICATION

For vaginal thrush take a tampon and dampen it then place 3 drops of *BLEND* on it and insert in the vagina for 2 hours.

Make up a bottle of Thrush Treatment Oil by adding 12 drops of *BLEND* to 30ml of Sweet Almond Oil. Apply the Treatment Oil night and morning to the affected area. Wear loose cotton pants and avoid wearing tights until the condition has cleared. Men whose sexual partners suffer from thrush should bathe their penis daily in a bowel of water to which 4 drops of *BLEND* have been added.

LIFE STYLE

Use sanitary pads not tampons for your periods. Don't take antibiotics unless absolutely necessary. Tell your doctor you are prone to thrush. Don't use strong detergents etc.

BATHS

Put 8 drops of *BLEND* in your bath. Soak and relax.

DIET

Cut out sugars and starches.
Eat natural yoghourts.
Take Garlic Tablets and Acidophilus as per container.

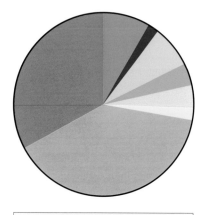

☐ esters	8.5%
■ aliphatic aldehydes	1.7%
☐ ketones	7.3%
☐ sesquiterpenes	3.8%
■ lactones and coumarins	trace
☐ remainder	4.2%
☐ oxides	2.3%
☐ acids	trace
■ aromatic aldehydes	
☐ monoterpenes	39.2%
■ alcohols	33.0%
■ phenols, phe.ethers	

CCP of BLEND RECIPE

  Cypress (cupressus sempervirens)

  Mint Peppermint (mentha piperita)

  Geranium (pelargonium graveolens)

Cypress is astringent, bactericidal and balances the sympathetic nerve system. It constricts blood vessels and is recommended for broken capillaries , cellulite, haemorrhoids, pyorrhea, rheumatism and sweaty feet.

Mint Peppermint antiinflammatory, bactericidal, an analgesic and a tonic to the system. It constricts capillaries and is recommended for asthma, eczema, gnats, herpes, rashes, ringworm and yellow fever.

Geranium is anticoagulant, bactericidal and a tonic. It constricts blood vessels, stems bleeding and is recommended for fluid retention and varicose veins. Traditionally a great healing plant often planted around dwellings to ward off evil spirits.

Chemical constituents to be found in the blend may include:

- ☐ α–terpinyl acetate, menthyl acetate citronellyl formate, geranyl formate
- ■ citral
- ☐ menthone, isomenthone, pulegone
- ☐ guaiazulene, β-caryophyllene, cedrene, cadinene, germacrene,
- ■ aesculetine, menthofuran

- ☐ *cis*-rose oxide, 1.8-cineole
- ▨ α–pinene, β–pinene, Δ3-carene, *p*-cymene, camphene, limonene phellandrene, menthene
- ▨ cedrol, α-terpineol, borneol, sabinol, manool, menthol, neomenthol, citronellol, geraniol, linalool

BLEND

21 drops *Cypress*
 7 drops *Mint Peppermint*
14 drops *Geranium*
42 drops *BLEND*

Make up your *BLEND* using the quantities above - store in a small dark glass bottle fitted with a dropper (see page 20).

AILMENT

This is a painful condition when the veins become distended and knotted. They often show clearly on the surface of the legs and can also form just inside the rectum - see under haemorrhoids.

Obstruction of the blood flow causing pressure on the veins is the cause of the damage. The valves in the veins become damaged and no longer function well. In the legs where the blood is flowing against gravity this results in the veins becoming knotted and distended.

Varicose veins can begin to develop as early as the teenage years. They occur frequently during pregnancy. People whose jobs involve many hours of standing are also at risk of this condition. Obesity also causes strain on the veins.

Phlebitis occurs if veins become inflamed and this sometimes results in a blood clot forming

TREATMENT

Once the vein is badly damaged it is not possible to repair it. However to help the circulation it is advised to wear support stockings.

Make up a bottle of Varicose Vein Treatment Oil by adding 12 drops of *BLEND* to 30ml of Sweet Almond Oil (see page 20).

Apply the Treatment Oil night and morning to the affected area. If working with the leg use strokes from the ankle to the thigh. Always work towards the heart as you are helping the veins send the blood back to the heart. Use the palm of your hand and not your fingers.

LIFE STYLE

To keep the condition under control avoid standing for long periods. If standing still, to help the blood flow, flex the leg muscles regularly. Take regular exercise. Do not cross your legs when sitting down.

COMPRESSES

To relieve the aching pain prepare cold compresses by adding 4 drops of *BLEND* to ice cold water. Use a cotton cloth, soak in the water, wring out and place around the area.

BATHS

Put 6 drops of *BLEND* in your bath. Soak and relax. Do not have your bath water too hot.

DIET

If necessary follow a weight reduction diet.
Supplements
Parsley and Garlic
Vitamin C, Vitamin E, Rutin, Lecithin

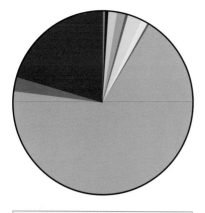

◼ esters	0.2%
◼ aliphatic aldehydes	0.6%
◻ ketones	1.7%
◼ sesquiterpenes	1.5%
◼ lactones and coumarins	0.2%
◻ remainder	3.4%
◻ oxides	1.0%
◻ acids	trace
◼ aromatic aldehydes	0.1%
◼ monoterpenes	68.0%
◼ alcohols	2.7%
◼ phenols, phe.ethers	20.6%

CCP of BLEND RECIPE

Fennel Sweet (foeniculum vulgare)

Juniper Berry (juniperus communis)

Grapefruit (citrus paradisi)

Fennel Sweet is a decongestant, antiinflammatory and diuretic. It is recommended for cellulite, dissolves boils and treats swellings, fluid retention, oedema and wrinkles. Avoid in cases of pregnancy or epilepsy.

Juniper Berry is diuretic and acts as a regulator. It is recommended for cellulite, fluid retention, obesity, oedema, painful joints, psoriasis, stiffness and it eliminates uric acid from the joints.

Grapefruit treats congested skin. It is calming and relieves stress headaches. It generally aids digestion. It is a diuretic and has a general cleansing effect on the body.

Chemical constituents to be found in the blend may include:

- ◼ geranyl acetate
- ◼ citronellal, citral, sinensal
- ◻ fenchone
- ◼ caryophyllene, cadinene, humulenes, germacrene, cadinene
- ◼ umbelliferone, auraptene, limettin bergaptene, umbelliferone
- ◻ 1.8-cineole, caryophyllene oxide
- ◻ anisic acid
- ◼ anisaldehyde
- ◼ α-pinene, α-thujene, γ-terpinene, limonene, myrcene, phellandrene p-cymene, sabinene, camphene
- ◼ fenchol, terpinen-4-ol, α-terpineol paradisiol, geraniol
- ◼ trans-anethole, methyl chavicol

BLEND

16 drops *Fennel Sweet*
12 drops *Juniper Berry*
20 drops *Grapefruit*
48 drops *BLEND*

Make up your *BLEND* using the quantities above - store in a small dark glass bottle fitted with a dropper (see page 20).

AILMENT

Obesity is the condition where the body has stored so much extra fat that health is threatened. Overweight can lead to various conditions such as high blood pressure, poor circulation, diabetes, gall bladder problems, gout, heart disorders, heart attacks and shortened life expectancy.

Over weight is caused by overeating in as much that more calories are being taken in than are being burnt up by the body. To adjust the fat level in the body a controlled food plan and life style need to be undertaken. Sometimes young girls are so driven to reduce weight that they cease to eat at all and are unable to reverse the process. This inability to eat diagnosed as anorexia is an extremely dangerous condition and needs expert advice. Help can be obtained from Maisner Centre for Eating Disorders, P.O. Box 464, Hove, East Sussex BN3 2BN.

TREATMENT

To tackle the problem of obesity individual treatment plans need to be developed. People have different metabolic rates which is one factor but emotional, psychological and social pressures all play a part. Seek out a friend or a local slimming group such as Weight Watchers to help you develop your own strategy. You will need to adopt a programme that you can establish as a life long pattern. Do not go for crash dieting - this can do more harm than good in the long term.

Essential oils can most certainly help to reduce fluid retention and also work on your metabolism and hormonal balance.

MASSAGE

Food is often turned to as a comfort. Replace it with a full body massage by booking regular appointments with an aromatherapist. They will also counsel you on your progress and provide another support in your strategy to establish a new life style. At home make up a bottle of Weight Loss Treatment Oil by adding 12 drops of *BLEND* to 30ml of Sweet Almond Oil (see page 20). Use your Treatment Oil, every day, to massage all around your shoulders and lower back. Get a friend to massage your back regularly.

BATHS

Put 8 drops of *BLEND* in your bath. Soak and relax.

DIET

Work out your controlled food plan with advice from an expert. Always include 8 glasses of spring water a day.

—Chemical Constituents Index—

◻ Esters

angelates 30, 34, 36, 38, 40, 48, 50, 64,
66, 98, 100, 102
benzyl acetate 42, 68, 90
benzyl benzoate 90
bornyl acetate 24, 44, 50, 58, 62, 70, 98,
100, 106
bornyl butyrate 24
butyrates 30, 34, 36, 38, 40, 48, 50, 64,
100
cis-carvyl acetate 74
cinnamyl acetate 90
citronellyl acetate 46, 58, 68, 102, 104,
112
citronellyl butyrate 82
citronellyl citronellate 82
citronellyl formate 98, 100, 120
fenchyl acetate 62, 70, 76
geranyl acetate 24, 26, 30, 42, 54, 58, 60,
66, 68, 70, 72, 76, 80, 82, 86, 90, 92,
94, 102, 104, 106, 108, 110, 112, 116,
118, 122
geranyl formate 120
lavandulyl acetate 32, 36, 46, 54, 62, 66,
70, 80, 82, 88, 96, 106, 110, 116, 118
linalyl acetate 24, 26, 28, 30, 32, 36, 42,
46, 52, 54, 58, 60, 62, 66, 68, 70, 74,
76, 80, 82, 86, 88, 92, 94, 96, 104,
106, 108, 110, 112, 116, 118
menthyl acetate 40, 80, 120
methyl anthranilate 34, 60, 92, 116
methyl cinnamate 62, 76
methyl myrtenate 50
myrrholic ester 84, 118
neryl acetate 24, 26, 92, 94, 98, 104, 108,
112
propionates 64
terpinen-4-yl acetate 96
terpinyl acetate 30, 42, 44, 52, 60, 62, 70,
80, 94
α-terpinyl acetate 78, 82, 96, 102, 120
tiglates 30, 34, 36, 38, 40, 48, 50, 64, 66,
98, 100, 102

◼ Aliphatic Aldehydes

2-butanal 78, 84, 118
caryophyllenal 92, 104, 108
citral 26, 30, 32, 34, 36, 42, 54, 58, 60,
62, 66, 68, 70, 72, 80, 82, 84, 90, 94,
96, 98, 100, 104, 106, 110, 112, 116,
118, 120, 122
citronellal 40, 46, 60, 62, 64, 82, 86, 90,
94, 96, 98, 114, 116, 122
decanal 116
decyl aldehyde 74, 86
geranial 38, 40, 64, 86, 96, 114
neral 40, 102
nonanal 94, 98
octanal 94
sinensal 90, 116, 122
undecanal 58

◻ Ketones

atlantone 56
camphor 28, 36, 44, 46, 50, 54, 58, 62,
66, 70, 74, 80, 82, 86, 92, 94, 96, 98,
100, 104, 106, 108, 110, 116, 118
carvone 58, 70, 72, 74, 84, 86, 94
cryptone 44, 62
curzerenone 78, 84, 118
dihydrocarvone 58, 108
fenchone 122
gingerone 38, 40, 64, 86, 96, 114
isoartemisia 98, 100, 106
isomenthone 80, 120
isopatchoulenone 52, 78
isopinocamphone 50
jasmone 92
menthone 56, 68, 74, 80, 82, 98, 100, 120
methyl isobutyl ketone 78, 84, 118
octanone 54, 62, 66, 70, 80, 94, 96, 110,
116, 118
patchoulenone 52, 78
pinocamphone 50
pinocarvone 30, 32, 34, 36, 38, 40, 48, 50,
56, 64, 66, 82, 98, 100, 102
piperitone 48, 58, 108
pulegone 80, 120

santalone 64, 96, 112
tagetenones 28, 72, 84
tagetone 28, 72, 84
thujone 44, 58, 70, 92, 98, 100, 104, 108

◼ Sesquiterpenes

aromadendrene 32, 48, 56, 82, 90, 94,
110, 118
α-bergamotene 94, 98
bisabolene 24, 58, 72, 76, 108
β-bisabolene 68, 94, 98, 104, 112
bourbonene 74, 92, 104, 108
α-bulnesene 78
cadinene 48, 50, 52, 56, 60, 62, 70, 78,
84, 88, 90, 102, 110, 118, 120, 122
caryophyllene 30, 34, 38, 40, 42, 46, 50,
52, 56, 60, 64, 72, 74, 78, 92, 98, 100,
102, 104, 106, 112, 118, 122
β-caryophyllene 24, 32, 36, 44, 48, 54, 58,
62, 66, 68, 70, 76, 80, 82, 88, 90, 96,
108, 110, 114, 116, 120
cedrene 24, 52, 78, 96, 102, 120
chamazulene 30, 34, 36, 38, 40, 46, 48,
50, 54, 60, 64, 66, 72, 98, 100, 102,
106
copaene 58, 62, 78, 84, 118
ar-curcumene 38, 40, 86, 114
curcumenes 64, 112
curzerene 84
daucene 72, 76
dihydroazulene 98, 100, 106
elemene 72, 74, 76, 78, 84, 88, 118
farnesene 38, 54, 58, 60, 62, 64, 66, 72,
74, 112
germacrene 24, 42, 50, 56, 68, 70, 80, 92,
98, 100, 104, 106, 108, 120, 122
guaiazulene 68, 120
guaiene 62
α-guaiene 52, 78
heerabolene 84, 118
humulenes 50, 52, 58, 70, 82, 108, 114,
122
lindestrene 84
patchoulenes 52, 78
santalenes 64, 96, 112

β-sesquiphellandrene 38, 40, 64, 86, 96,
114
seychellenes 78
thujopsene 24
viridiflorene 32, 48, 90, 94, 110, 118
zingiberene 38, 40, 64, 86, 96, 114

◼ Lactones and Coumarins

achilline 98, 100, 106
aesculetine 80, 120
auraptene 90, 122
bergamottin 94, 98
bergaptene 42, 68, 74, 86, 94, 98, 104,
112, 122
coumarin 32, 36, 46, 54, 62, 66, 70, 80,
82, 94, 96, 106, 110, 116, 118
indole 92
limettin 90, 122
menthofuran 80, 120
umbelliferone 50, 54, 62, 66, 70, 74, 82,
86, 94, 96, 106, 110, 116, 118, 122

☐ Remainder

cis-spiro-ether 54, 60, 66, 72, 106
damascenone 26, 102, 104, 112
en-yn-dicycloether 54, 60, 66, 72, 106

☐ Oxides

α-bisabolol oxide 38, 46, 54, 60, 66, 72,
106
bulnesene oxide 52, 78
1.4-cineole 90
caryophyllene oxide 50, 52, 54, 58, 66, 70,
78, 80, 82, 92, 96, 108, 114, 122
1.8-cineole 24, 28, 30, 32, 34, 36, 38, 40,
44, 46, 48, 50, 52, 54, 56, 58, 62, 64,
66, 70, 74, 76, 78, 80, 82, 86, 90, 92,
94, 96, 98, 100, 102, 104, 106, 108,
110, 114, 116, 118, 120, 122
guaiene oxide 52, 78
humulene oxide 44, 114
linalool oxide 54, 62, 66, 70, 94, 96, 110,
116, 118

manoyl oxide 52, 96, 102
rose oxide 26, 102, 104, 112
cis-rose oxide 68, 98, 100, 120

☐ Acids

anisic acid 122
myrrholic acid 78, 84, 118
nortricycloekasantalic acid 64, 96, 112
phenylacetic acid 92
valeric acid 72

◼ Aromatic Aldehydes

anisaldehyde 122
benzaldehyde 46, 54, 62, 66, 70, 80, 82,
    94, 96, 106, 110, 116
benzyl aldehyde 36
cinnamaldehyde 78, 84, 90, 118
cuminaldehyde 36, 46, 54, 62, 66, 70, 78,
    80, 82, 84, 94, 96, 106, 110, 116, 118
methyl vanillin 90
piperonal 58
salicylaldehyde 72, 84

☐ Monoterpenes

camphene 38, 48, 50, 54, 58, 64, 70, 72,
    74, 76, 78, 84, 86, 96, 98, 100, 102,
    104, 106, 108, 110, 112, 114, 118, 120,
    122
Δ3-carene 78, 96, 102, 120
p-cymene 28, 30, 32, 34, 42, 48, 50, 52,
    58, 60, 70, 76, 78, 80, 82, 86, 88, 90,
    94, 96, 98, 102, 110, 114, 116, 118,
    120, 122
dipentene 78
limonene 24, 26, 28, 30, 34, 40, 42, 44,
    48, 50, 52, 54, 58, 60, 62, 64, 68, 70,
    72, 74, 76, 78, 80, 82, 84, 86, 90, 92,
    94, 96, 98, 100, 102, 104, 106, 108,
    110, 112, 114, 116, 118, 120, 122
menthene 120
myrcene 24, 26, 30, 34, 42, 44, 50, 52, 58,
    60, 62, 70, 72, 80, 84, 92, 94, 98, 100,
    108, 110, 114, 116, 118, 122

ocimene 28, 30, 42, 54, 58, 60, 70, 80, 84,
    102, 106, 110, 116, 118
cis-ocimene 62, 76
phellandrene 58, 64, 74, 92, 108, 120, 122
α-phellandrene 48
α-pinene 24, 26, 28, 32, 34, 36, 38, 40,
    42, 44, 46, 48, 50, 52, 58, 62, 64, 68,
    70, 72, 74, 76, 78, 80, 82, 86, 88, 90,
    92, 94, 96, 98, 100, 102, 106, 108,
    110, 114, 118, 120, 122
β-pinene 24, 26, 30, 38, 42, 44, 50, 52,
    58, 60, 62, 64, 68, 72, 74, 76, 78, 80,
    86, 88, 92, 96, 98, 100, 102, 104, 106,
    108, 112, 114, 120
pinenes 84, 116
sabinene 30, 36, 42, 44, 50, 52, 58, 60,
    62, 64, 70, 80, 94, 98, 100, 106, 108,
    114, 122
stearoptene 26, 102, 104, 112
α-terpinene 26, 28, 30, 32, 42, 48, 52, 60,
    68, 74, 80, 88, 90, 94, 104, 110, 112,
    114, 118
γ-terpinene 26, 28, 30, 32, 34, 42, 44, 48,
    50, 52, 60, 68, 70, 74, 76, 80, 86, 88,
    90, 94, 98, 104, 110, 112, 114, 116,
    118, 122
terpinenes 108
terpinolene 28, 32, 90, 94, 110, 118
thujene 48, 50, 70, 108
α-thujene 122

◼ Alcohols

artemisia alcohol 24
atlantol 56
benzyl alcohol, 92
α-bisabolol 38, 46, 54, 60, 66, 72, 92,
    106, 108
borneol 32, 40, 44, 46, 50, 54, 58, 60, 62,
    64, 66, 70, 74, 78, 80, 82, 86, 88, 90,
    94, 96, 106, 110, 112, 114, 116, 118,
    120
bulnesol 52, 78
cadinol 106
carotol 76
cedrol 24, 52, 56, 78, 96, 120

citronellol 26, 34, 38, 40, 46, 58, 64, 68,
 76, 82, 86, 98, 100, 102, 104, 112,
 114, 116, 120
daucol 76
γ-eudesmol 24
farnesol 30, 34, 36, 48, 64, 66, 68, 100,
 104, 112
fenchol 122
geraniol 24, 26, 50, 54, 66, 68, 70, 74, 76,
 80, 86, 88, 90, 92, 94, 96, 98, 100,
 102, 104, 106, 112, 114, 116, 120, 122
gingerol 38, 40, 64, 86, 96, 114
globulol 24, 32, 48, 56, 90, 110
guaiol 52, 78
lavandulol 32, 36, 46, 54, 62, 66, 70, 80,
 82, 88, 94, 96, 106, 110, 116, 118
linalool 24, 26, 28, 30, 34, 36, 38, 40, 42,
 44, 48, 50, 52, 54, 58, 60, 62, 64, 66,
 68, 70, 72, 74, 76, 80, 82, 84, 86, 88,
 90, 92, 94, 96, 98, 100, 104, 106, 108,
 110, 112, 114, 116, 118, 120
manool 52, 120
menthol 56, 74, 80, 120
myrrh alcohols 78, 84, 88, 118
neomenthol 80, 120
nerol 26, 40, 58, 92, 102, 104, 112
nerolidol 48, 64, 66, 92, 100
octanol 116
paradisiol 90, 122
patchouli alcohols 52, 78
phenylethyl alcohol 26, 92
pinocarveol 56
trans-pinocarveol 48, 50, 64, 66, 102
piperitol 48
pogostol 52, 78
sabinol 52, 78, 96, 102, 120
santalols 64, 96, 112
santolina alcohol, 24
sclareol 42, 92, 104, 108
terpinen-4-ol 28, 30, 32, 36, 42, 44, 46,
 48, 50, 54, 58, 60, 62, 66, 70, 76, 80,
 82, 88, 90, 94, 96, 106, 108, 110, 114,
 118, 122

α-terpineol 24, 26, 28, 30, 32, 34, 36, 38,
 40, 42, 46, 48, 50, 52, 54, 58, 60, 62,
 64, 66, 70, 74, 76, 78, 80, 82, 86, 88,
 90, 92, 94, 96, 100, 102, 104, 106,
 108, 110, 116, 118, 120, 122
tricycloekasantalol 64, 112
viridiflorol 24, 48, 110
widdrol 24
yomogi alcohol 24

∎ Phenols and phen. ethers

aceteugenol 44, 82, 90, 108, 114
anethole 74, 86, 94
trans-anethole 122
asarone 72, 76
carvacrol 44, 52, 60, 80
elemicin 114
eugenol 44, 60, 62, 68, 76, 78, 80, 82, 84,
 90, 98, 100, 106, 108, 114, 116, 118
isoeugenol 82, 114
methyl chavicol (estragole) 50, 62, 76,
 122
methyl eugenol 42, 76, 102, 104, 112
methyl hexyl ether 92, 104, 108
myristicin 108, 114
safrole 68, 90, 108, 114
thymol 44, 52, 60, 116

Bibliography

British Herbal Pharmacopoeia, British Herbal Medicine Association, 1983.

Culpeper, N., Culpeper's Complete Herbal, W. Foulsham and Co. Ltd, 1952.

Davis, P., Aromatherapy An A-Z, C.W.Daniel, 1988.

Franchomme, P., Livre Quatrième, Eléments de Matière Médicale Aromatique Fondamentale.

Franchomme, P., Phytoguide I, International Phytomedical Foundation, La Courtête, France, 1985.

Franchomme, P. and Pénoël, D., L'Aromathérapie Exactement, 1990.

Grieve, M., A Modern Herbal, Penguin, 1982.

Grosjean, N., Aromatherapy from Provence, C.W.Daniel, 1993.

Guenther, E., The Essential Oils, Vol. 1-6., Van Nostrand, New York, 1948.

Jackson, J., Aromatherapy, Dorling Kindersley, 1987.

Lis-Balchin, M., The Chemistry and Bioactivity of Essential Oils, Amberwood, 1995.

Lawless, J., The Encyclopaedia of Essential Oils, Element Books, 1992.

Lawless, J., Aromatherapy and the Mind, Thorsons,1994.

Lawrence, B.M. Essential Oils, Allured Publishing Co., Wheaton, USA, 1978.

Kroch, A.&C.A., Guide to the Medicinal Plants of the United States, Quadrangle, The New York Times Book Co., 1973.

Mabey, R.(Ed.), The Complete New Herbal, Elm Tree Books, London, !988.

Maury, M., Marguerite Maury's Guide to Aromatherapy, C.W. Daniel, 1989.

Mills, S.Y., The Essential Book Of Herbal Medicine, Penguin Arkana, Harmonsworth.

Metcalfe, J., Herbs and Aromatherapy, Webb and Bower, 1989.

Phillips, R., Wild Flowers of Britain, Pan, 1977.

Ody, P., The Herb Society's Complete Medicinal Herbal, 1992.

Percival, A., Aromatherapy-A Nurse's Guide, Amberwood,1991.

Price, S., Aromatherapy for Common Ailments, Gaia Books, 1991.

Price, S., Aromatherapy Workbook, Thorsons, 1992.

Price, S. and Price, L., Aromatherapy for Health Professionals, Churchill Livingstone, 1995.

Ranson, F., British Herbs, Penguin, 1949.

Rich, P., Practical Aromatherapy, Parragon Book Services, 1994.

Ryman, D. The Aromatherapy Handbook, Century, 1984.

Secondi, O., Handbook of Perfumes and Flavors, Chemical Publishing Co., New York, 1990.

Sellar, W., The Directory of Essential Oils, C.W.Daniel, 1992.

Stead, C., The Power of Holistic Aromatherapy, Javelin Books, 1986.

Le Strange, R., A History of Herbal Plants, Angus and Robertson, 1977.

Tisserand, M., Aromatherapy for Women, Thorsons, 1990.

Tisserand, M., Stress: The Aromatic Solution, Hodder and Stoughton, 1996.

Tisserand, R. and Balacs, T., Essential Oil Safety, A Guide for Health Care Professionals, Churchill Livingstone, 1995.

Valnet, J., The Practice of Aromatherapy, C.W. Daniel (English Version), 1982.

Westwood, C., Aromatherapy-A Guide for Home Use, Amberwood, 1991.

Westwood, C., Aromatherapy-For Stress Management, Amberwood, 1991.

Wildwood, C., Aromatherapy, Element Books, 1991.

Worwood, V.A., The Fragrant Pharmacy, Macmillan, 1990.

Worwood, V.A., The Fragrant Mind, Doubleday, 1990.

Appendix

Thomas Holmes and Richard Rahe, two stress experts, produced the following way to check out stress levels. To rate yourself on the scale, add up the scores for all the listed events that you have experienced in the last year. If your total exceeds 150 there is a 50% chance that your health will be affected. A score of over 300 and there is a 90% chance that your health will be affected.

Use the scores to help plan a life style that will avoid facing too many stressful events simultaneously.

Death of spouse	100
Divorce	73
Marital separation	65
Jail term	63
Death of close family member	63
Personal injury or illness	53
Marriage	50
Loss of job	47
Marital reconciliation	45
Retirement	45
Change in health of family member	44
Pregnancy	40
Sexual problems	39
Gain of family member	39
Business readjustment	39
Change in financial state	38
Death of close friend	37
Change to a different type of work	36
Change in number of arguments with spouse	35
High mortgage	31
Foreclosure of mortgage or loan	30
Change in responsibility at work	29
Son or daughter leaving home	29
Trouble with in-laws	29
Outstanding personal achievement	28
Spouse begins or stops work	26
Beginning or ending education	26
Change in living conditions	25
Change in personal habits	24
Trouble with the boss	23
Change in working hours or conditions	20
Moving house	20
Changing schools	20
Change in leisure pursuits	19
Change in church activities	19
Change in social activities	18
Low to medium mortgage or loan	17
Altered sleeping habits	16
Change in number of family get-togethers	15
Change in eating habits	15
Going on holiday	13
Approaching Christmas season	12
Minor violations of the law	11

OTHER BOOKS AVAILABLE FROM AMBERWOOD PUBLISHING ARE:

AROMATHERAPY - *A guide for home use* by Christine Westwood. All you need to know about essential oils and using them.
£1.99   ISBN 0 9517723 0 9.

AROMATHERAPY - STRESS MANAGEMENT - *A guide for home use* by Christine Westwood. Covering the use of essential oils for everyday stress-related problems.
£3.50   ISBN 0 9517723 6 8.

AROMATHERAPY - FOR HEALTHY LEGS & FEET - *A guide for home use* by Christine Westwood. A guide to the home use of essential oils for the treatment of legs and feet.
£2.99   ISBN 1 899308 02 4.

AROMATHERAPY - A NURSES GUIDE by Ann Percival SRN. The ultimate safe lay guide to the natural benefits of Aromatherapy. Including recipes and massage techniques for many medical conditions and a quick reference chart.
£2.99   ISBN 1 899308 04 0.

AROMATHERAPY - A NURSES GUIDE FOR WOMEN by Ann Percival SRN. Concentrates on women's health for all ages. Including sections on PMT, menopause, infertility and cellulite.
£2.99   ISBN 1 899308 12 1.

AROMATHERAPY - ESSENTIAL OILS IN COLOUR by Rosemary Caddy Bsc Hons, ARCS MISPA. Exploring the chemistry of pure essential oils in colour gives the ancient art of Aromatherapy a completely new twist. A "must" for qualified aromatherapists, students and new converts alike.
£9.99   ISBN 1 899308 14 8.

AROMATHERAPY LEXICON - *The Essential Reference* by Geoff Lyth and Sue Charles. This informative Lexicon is remarkable for its simplicity and makes understanding Aromatherapy easy. This form of reference will give endless pleasure to beginners as well as practised Aromatherapists.
£4.99   ISBN 1 899308 15 6.

AROMATHERAPY - SIMPLY FOR YOU by Marion Del Gaudio Mak. A new updated edition of the simple and thorough guide to Aromatherapy that has been so successful. Easy reference chapters explain everything from purchasing and storage of essential oils to the beneficial effects to be had from their use.
£2.99   ISBN 1 899308 10 5.

AROMATHERAPY - THE CHEMISTRY & BIOACTIVITY OF ESSENTIAL OILS by Dr Maria Lis-Balchin. With a comprehensive list of the Oils and scientific analyses. Includes a section on the sense of smell and the history of Aromatherapy.
£5.99   ISBN 1 899308 21 0.

ALL YOU EVER WANTED TO KNOW ABOUT VITAMINS by Dr. Leonard Mervyn. Dr Mervyn explains why we need extra vitamins, and what can happen to our long term health if we don't get them in adaquate quantities, and who is most at risk from deficiency.
£6.99   ISBN 1 899308 22 9.

INDIAN MEDICINE - FOR THE IMMUNE SYSTEM - *Echinacea by Dr Desmond Corrigan* BSc(Pharms), MA, Phd, FLS, FPSI. An intriguing account of the history of the plant called Echinacea and its power to influence the immune system.
£2.99   ISBN 0 9517723 7 6.

HERBAL MEDICINE FOR SLEEP AND RELAXATION *by Dr Desmond Corrigan* BSc(Pharms), MA, Phd, FLS, FPSI. A guide to the natural sedatives as an alternitive to orthodox drug therapies, drawing on the latest medical research, presented in an easy reference format.
£2.99   ISBN 1 899308 07 5.

GINKGO BILOBA - ANCIENT MEDICINE *by Dr Desmond Corrigan* BSc(Pharms), MA, Phd, FLS, FPSI. (New Edition) Improved memory, circulation and concentration are associated with Ginko Biloba and explained in this book.
£2.99   ISBN 1 899308 04 0.

NATURAL TASTE - HERBAL TEAS - *A guide for home use by Andrew Chevallier* BA, MNIMH. Contains an impressive compendium of Herbal Teas gives information on how to make it, its benefits, history and folklore.
£3.50   ISBN 0 9517723 8 4.

NATURAL MEDICINE - HERBAL FIRST AID - *A guide for home use by Andrew Chevallier* BA, MNIMH. A beautifully clear reference book of natural remedies and general first aid in the home.
£2.99   ISBN 0 9517723 5 X.

PLANT MEDICINE - *A guide for home use by Charlotte Mitchell* MNIMH (New Edition).This book provides the perfect guide, explaining both the properties of plant medicines and how to use them. As more and more people seek alternatives to modern drugs, interest in natural plant remedies grows.
£2.99   ISBN 1 899308 13 X.

HOW GARLIC PROTECTS YOUR HEART *by Professor Edzard Ernst* MD PhD. Used as a medicine for over 4500 years, this book examines the latest scientific evidence supporting Garlic's effect in reducing cardiovascular disease, the Western World's number one killer.
£3.99   ISBN 1 899308 08 3.

WOMEN MEDICINE - VITEX AGNUS-CASTUS *by Simon Mills* MA, FNIMH. The story of the herb that has been used for centuries in the treatment of women's problems. The author examines the medical properties on symptoms relating to menstruation and the menopause.
£2.99   ISBN 0 9517723 3 3.

FENG SHUI - *A guide for home use by Karen Ward*. Simple tips on 'Power of Place' and effects of environment on health.
£2.99   ISBN 1 8993082 3 7.

INSOMNIA - DOCTOR I CAN'T SLEEP *by Dr Andrian Williams* FRCS. Written by one of the worlds sleep experts, Dr Williams explains the phenomenon of sleep and sleeping disorders and gives advice on treatment. With 25% of the adult population reporting difficulties sleeping - this book is essential reading for many.
£2.99   ISBN 1 899308 09 1.

ARTHRITIS & RHEUMATISM - *The Sufferers Guide by Dr John Cosh* FRCP MD. It is a complete guide to understanding the painful and sometimes progressive disease, whilst offering many useful tips to alleviate the symptoms.
£4.95   ISBN 1 899308 17 2.

SIGNS AND SYMPTOMS OF VITAMIN DEFICIENCY *by Dr Leonard Mervyn.* A simply written guide that will enable the lay reader to recognise and interpret vitamin deficiencies. Leonard Mervyn is a world renowned expert in dietary supplements and vitamins and minerals.
£2.99   ISBN 1 899308 06 7.

CAUSES AND PREVENTION OF VITAMIN DEFICIENCY *by Dr Leonard Mervyn.* A simply written guide that will enable the lay reader to take action to correct vitamin deficiences. A companion book to SIGNS AND SYMPTOMS OF VITAMIN DEFICIENCES.
£2.99   ISBN 1 899308 11 3.

VITAMINS ABC & OTHER FOOD FACTS *by Eileen Palmer.* This excellently illustrated book is designed both to encourage healthy eating and to make learning about vitamins, minerals and nutrition, fun.
£3.99   ISBN 0 9517723 2 5.

EYE CARE EYE WEAR - FOR BETTER VISION *by Mark Rossi* BSc, MBCO. A complete guide to eye care and eye wear including an assessment of the types of spectacles and contact lenses available and the latest corrective surgical procedures.
£3.99   ISBN 1 899308 01 6.

AROMATHERAPY - THE BABY BOOK *by Marion Del Gaudio Mak.* An easy to follow guide to massage for the infant or child.
£3.99   ISBN 1 899308 18 0.

AROMATHERAPY THE PREGNANCY BOOK *by Jennie Supper* RM RN MGCP. Midwife Jennie Supper has many years experience of bringing new people into the world. Her book deals with making the birthing process pleasurable by using beautiful aromas for calming tension and natural pain relief.
£5.99   ISBN 1 899308 20 2.

PHYTOTHERAPY 50 VITAL HERBS *by Andrew Chevallier.* The most popular medicinal herbs with uses and advice written by an expert.
£6.99   ISBN 1 899308 19 9.

ESSENTIAL OILS IN COLOUR

• AROMATHERAPY •

Essential Oils in Colour
CADDY CLASSIC PROFILES

• Rosemary Caddy •
BSc Hons ARCS MISPA

- *Aromatherapy in Living Colour*
- *Chemistry at a Glance*
- *Comprehensive Index*
- *Enables Creative Blending*
- *90 Classic Profiles*

ISBN 1-899308-14-8

Readers Review:

Summary : A completely new approach to understanding essential oils.

This exciting and original book will be useful to all interested in essential oils. The author has developed a logical system of profiling the oils. This clearly structured visual system makes it possible to see at a glance the qualities of each essential oil.

The book devotes a complete page to each oil. The percentage of each chemical family present in the oil is given; this is also presented visually by means of a piechart. All the reported therapeutic properties of the oil are covered. Finally the major individual chemical constituents to be found in the oil are listed.

I found this book excellent for comparing essential oils and in choosing which oils to blend to help clients with specific problems.

It will also be useful to those interested in understanding and using essential oils to treat common ailments in the home.

It is a unique contribution to any aromatherapy book shelf.

Amberwood Publishing Limited, Rochester, England
Phone: 01634 290115 or Fax: 01634 290761
E-mail: books@amberwoodpublishing.com   Website: www.amberwoodpublishing.com

Blending Example

CADDY BLENDING CALCULATOR

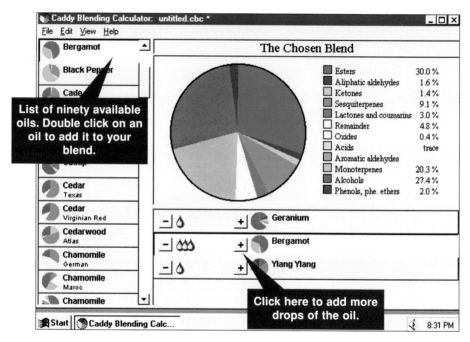

- *Enables Creative Blending*
- *90 Essential Oils to Blend*
- *Step by Step Instructions*
- *Blends in Living Colour*
- *Make-up of Blend at a Glance*
- *Print on Client's Record Sheet*

An excellent companion to both 'Essential Oils in Colour' and 'The Essential Blending Guide' the Caddy Blending Calculator opens up a new world of exploration. At a glance you can see the chemical make-up of any blend.

You can explore your trusted blends and see their chemical make-up. You can adjust your blends to suit individual needs. Print your blend for your records.

Windows 95/98

October Pen SOFTWARE

CD-ROM

For further information:
E-mail: mail@ccprofiles.co.uk   Website: www.ccprofiles.co.uk

Teaching Materials

Essential Oils in Colour

Caddy Blending Calculator

The Essential Blending Guide - 50 Common Ailments

Teaching Packs - available to Schools

For further information:
E-mail: mail@ccprofiles.co.uk   Website: www.ccprofiles.co.uk

Materials for Tutors and Students

Caddy Profiles Course Pack
Teaching Pack 1

Chapter 1 : Concept of Caddy Profiles
Chapter 2 : Chemical Families
Chapter 3 : Comparing Essential Oils
Chapter 4 : Blending Essential Oils
Chapter 5 : Case Study

Caddy Chemistry Course Pack
Teaching Pack 2

Chapter 1 : Elements and Atomic Structure
Chapter 2 : Compounds and Molecules
Chapter 3 : Essential Oil Molecules

In both Course Packs the course documentaton consists of a Tutor's Pack and a Student's Pack.
The Student's pack is a workbook which is completed during the course.
The Tutor's Pack contains detailed lecturing notes together with full solutions for the student's worksheets. Masters for OHP's are included.

Chemical Families
Student Pack 1
Monoterpenes
Sesquiterpenes
Alcohols
Phenols
Aldehydes
Acids
Esters
Ketones
Phenolic Ethers
Oxides
Lactones and Coumarins

This set of 11 sheets is taken from the Chemistry Course Pack, and may be of interest to individual students and other users of the books or software

For further information:
E-mail: mail@ccprofiles.co.uk   Website: www.ccprofiles.co.uk